A distinguished team of contributors from the fields of medicine, philosophy, and law addresses some of the pressing issues which arise over the provision of care for dependent elderly patients. Some of the chapters are concerned with the challenge of achieving good quality medical care, the chronic inadequacies of policy making in the UK context, and the prospects for improvement in the medium term. Other chapters look at some of the threats to dependent elderly patients posed by longer term social and ideological trends which find expression in proposals for age-limits to health care, advocacy of living wills and euthanasia, arguments for withdrawing tube-feeding from certain categories of patient, and certain proposals for resource allocation. This interdisciplinary volume will have a wide appeal to those involved in care of the dependent elderly, to health policy analysts and health care economists, and to bioethicists.

The dependent elderly

THE DEPENDENT ELDERLY: AUTONOMY, JUSTICE AND QUALITY OF CARE

Edited by

LUKE GORMALLY

Director
The Linacre Centre for Health Care Ethics

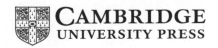

CAMBRIDGE
UNIVERSITY PRESS

Published by the Press Syndicate at the University of Cambridge
The Pitt Building, Trumpington Street, Cambridge CB2 1RP
40 West 20th Street, New York, NY 10011–4211, USA
10 Stamford Road, Oakleigh, Victoria 3166, Australia

First published 1992

Printed in Great Britain at the University Press, Cambridge

A catalogue record for this book is available from the British Library

Library of Congress cataloguing in publication data

The Dependent elderly: autonomy, justice, and quality of care / edited by Luke Gormally.
    p.   cm.
ISBN 0–521–41531–4 (hardback)
1. Frail elderly – Medical care.   I. Gormally, Luke.
[DNLM: 1. Health Services for the Aged.   2. Long-Term Care – in old age.
3. Quality of Health Care.   4. Quality of Life.   WT   30   D419]
RA564.8.D46   1992
362.1'9897–dc20
DNLM/DLC
for Library of Congress   92–4099   CIP

ISBN 0 521 41531 4 hardback

CE

Contents

Contributors

Michael Banner	Dean and Director of Studies in Philosophy and Theology, Peterhouse, Cambridge
Joseph Boyle	Professor of Philosophy and Principal, St Michael's College, University of Toronto
John Finnis	Professor of Law and Legal Philosophy, University of Oxford
Luke Gormally	Director, The Linacre Centre for Health Care Ethics, London
Marion Hildick-Smith	Consultant Physician in Geriatric Medicine, Nunnery Fields Hospital, Canterbury; President, British Geriatrics Society
Michael Horan	Professor of Geriatric Medicine, University of Manchester
David J Hunter	Director, Nuffield Institute for Health Services Studies, University of Leeds
John Keown	Director, Centre for Health Care Law, University of Leicester
Graham Mulley	Professor of Medicine for the Elderly, St James's University Hospital, Leeds
Robert Stout	Professor of Geriatric Medicine and Dean of The Faculty of Medicine, The Queen's University of Belfast

1

Introduction

LUKE GORMALLY

All the chapters in the present volume are based on papers which were originally delivered at two related Conferences planned by the editor for the 1990 Meeting of the European Association of Centres of Medical Ethics.[1] Most have been revised in the light of the responses to them at that Meeting.

Both Conferences were concerned with certain of the major ethical issues which arise in relation to the care of the dependent elderly, namely those old people whose condition is such that they require continuing care. It was decided to consider those issues principally as they present themselves in the context of UK Geriatric Medicine, though attention was also devoted to certain influential trends in the USA and The Netherlands.

The speciality of Geriatric Medicine has developed remarkably in the UK since the Second World War and is characterised, in the persons of so many of its practitioners, by a high degree of expertise and by admirable commitment to the health care of elderly people. These features of clinical practice of themselves are cause for hope in face of the increasing need for that expertise and commitment coming from the growing population of the dependent elderly. But realism demands that we should recognise the threats posed to the position of the dependent elderly in our society both by trends in social policy and by ideological trends. Some of the latter, if given expression in social and health care policy, would present a radical threat to the position of the dependent elderly in our society. A number of the papers in the present volume are concerned to confront those ideological trends as they find expression in proposals for age-limits to health care, in the advocacy of living wills and euthanasia, in arguments for withdrawing tube-feeding from certain categories of patient, and in specific proposals for resource allocation. Other papers identify the challenge of achieving good quality care of the dependent elderly, the chronic inadequacies of policy-making in that field, and the prospects in the medium term given current policy.

The issues on which the Conferences focussed are summarily named in the subtitle of the present volume: autonomy, justice and quality of care. Autonomy, properly understood, is an entirely admirable moral objective. But the notion of autonomy is employed in the advocacy of causes inimical to genuine respect for the dignity of the dependent elderly and corrosive of commitment to their care. Quality of care in the present volume is perceived as an issue of justice. The concerns which the idea of justice is intended to capture over the range of the following chapters are various:

> that in the ordering of society's affairs we should seek to obviate conditions which present a threat to the dignity of the most vulnerable members of society. It is that kind of concern which demands that we provide good quality of care for the dependent elderly.
>
> That everyone should refrain from choosing to act in ways which are incompatible with decent treatment of other human beings. This concern excludes abusing the dependent elderly, deliberately abandoning them when the resources exist to help them, and in the extreme killing them.
>
> And that we should avoid behaving in ways which have unfair consequences for others, even though what we choose to do is not precisely aimed at imposing those consequences on those who find themselves unfairly dealt with. This concern would exclude, for example, resource allocation policies the predictable consequences of which would be unfair to the dependent elderly.

Given the varied character of the concerns of justice identified here, the entire volume could be said to be about justice in the care of the dependent elderly.

Less evident in the content of the volume is the concern with autonomy, though it is an explicit concern of Professor Horan's paper and my own paper on the ethical framework of the Report on *The Living Will*, and is central in the apologetics for euthanasia as practised in The Netherlands (the subject of Dr Keown's paper) and as advocated in the UK and elsewhere.

The concept of autonomy is indeed so rhetorically attractive that it is employed in advancing ethical positions which are quite incompatible. Not surprisingly, therefore, it is associated with a good deal of confusion.

It might be useful, in this introduction, to cut a path through the contemporary jungle of talk about 'patient autonomy' and 'respect for patient autonomy'. Some may be grateful for the path though, doubtless, others will have plotted other routes. I shall first say something about autonomy in general and then something more particular about patient autonomy.

Autonomy in general

The words 'autonomy' and 'autonomous' are used in respect of a capacity, a condition and a right.

To be autonomous, as the word implies, is to be 'self-governed' or self-directed in the conduct of one's life; that is the condition. 'Autonomy' is used of the *capacity* to be self-directed in the conduct of one's life. 'Respect for autonomy' involves respect at least for this capacity. People speak of a 'right to autonomy' which demands respect. A right to autonomy must be a right to at least *some* exercise of the capacity for self-direction in one's life. But what exercise of that capacity? The answer we give to that question must surely depend on the understanding we have of the value of autonomy.

Some semi-popular talk about autonomy and the right to have one's autonomy respected seems to suggest that what people value is doing what they want (in the sense of acting on the wants, wishes and desires they *happen* to have) as distinct from having to do what someone else wants.

But it seems fairly clear that the ability to do what one *happens* to want to do is not sufficient for 'self-government' in the conduct of one's life. Someone whose condition is one of wanton self-indulgence does what he happens to want to do. What is valued in the capacity for self-government is at the very least our ability to evaluate our desires and to act selectively in accordance with our evaluations.

But will action in accordance with *any* kind of evaluation count as an exercise of autonomy? Our answer to this question will depend on what we think the point of self-government or self-direction is.

The capacity for self-government is properly exercised and developed with a view to the flourishing or well-being of the person who possesses it (a well-being which includes friendship and justice in community). If so exercised it is indeed an aspect of that flourishing. In what way is it an aspect?

Human happiness or well-being is not left to be wholly a matter of luck, or of grace which does not require willing cooperation; what we make of ourselves (in other words, our character) makes a big difference to whether or not we flourish as human beings. And our characters are decisively shaped by our chosen actions: these do not merely bring about effects external to us, they also serve to form our dispositions. Thus, if I choose to lie to someone I may or may not deceive that person, but I will certainly reinforce in myself the disposition to be a liar.

So choice and acting on choice are fundamental to the formation of character, and to the influence on human well-being or human misery that character has. A person's exercise of choice will in this way inescapably make for well-being or misery in his or her own life.

Now there is a clear case for valuing human choice, and so for valuing the exercise of autonomy, precisely in so far as it serves to form in us those dispositions which are conducive to human flourishing.

People differ in their views on how wide an exercise of the capacity for self-direction should be respected. One very important factor in determining those differing views is whether or not one believes there is human knowledge of moral truths, in particular knowledge of the objective requirements we need to meet if we are to flourish as human beings.

If there is such knowledge, then it is clear why we should value the exercise of choice in conformity with that knowledge: for evidently that would be an exercise of autonomy which makes for human flourishing. But it would not be obvious why we should value exercises of autonomy at variance with the objective requirements of human flourishing.

Still, if there is to be choice one has to allow not just for the possibility but also for the reality of erroneous choices. So, necessarily, respect for autonomy must leave scope for *some* erroneous choices. But it does not follow that any and every exercise of choice is to be respected. We need to bear in mind why this capacity is to be valued; and if our choices seriously undermine in us the capacity to flourish as human beings there is no reason of moral principle why those choices should be respected.

The two previous paragraphs explain what may be held to follow for our understanding of respect for autonomy from the belief that there is human knowledge of moral truths. But it is evident that many people in our society hold no such clear belief. For that minority who are seriously sceptical about the existence of *any* moral truths, there will be no reason to believe the claim that one should respect people's autonomy. For that much larger body of opinion which holds that morality essentially rests on subjective preferences ('Abortion may be wrong for you but I don't think it is.'), talk about respect for autonomy suggests the following: if people are not permitted to do what they want, it cannot be because of truly objective constraints, since they do not exist; it must be because of constraints imposed by the more or less arbitrary exercise of power.

The favourite 'theory' in our society about constraints on the exercise of autonomy maintains that such constraints are reasonable precisely in so far as they prevent 'harms' to third parties; what people choose to do to themselves or to consenting partners ('private choices') should not be the subject of constraints. But there is an element of arbitrariness about the theory. For if in talking about 'harms' we are to assume knowledge of the objective conditions of human flourishing, and if autonomy is to be valued just in so far as it makes for human flourishing, then why should we respect deeply harmful 'private choices' (choices by which people make themselves vicious)? But if we disclaim knowledge of the objective conditions of human flourishing, what entitles us to identify anything as 'harmful'?

Patient autonomy

What people understand by patient autonomy in our society is as varied as the understandings of autonomy in general.

Some who talk about patient autonomy primarily have in mind a right: the competent patient's right to decide about his or her medical treatment on the basis of adequate information and to have that right respected without fear of coercive pressures.

It is perfectly possible to find a place for a version of such a right within a traditional understanding of morality. It is notable that the early development of theological reflection from the fifteenth century about when life-prolonging treatment was to be regarded as ethically mandatory ('ordinary') and when it might be blamelessly refused (i.e. when it might be judged 'extraordinary') took place in response to questions raised by patients about *their* responsibilities in the matter. The assumption behind the way the answers were framed was that responsibility for decisions about health care properly and ultimately lay with the competent patient. The responsibility was thought to lie with the patient, first because health is a personal good, an aspect of our well-being or flourishing as human persons, for which each of us needs to assume responsibility. But the extent to which each person can afford to cultivate his or her health (or attend to its restoration) must depend on that person's other commitments, so that is a second reason why responsibility for health care decisions must ultimately lie with the competent patient.

There is, then, a context of traditional ethical reflection in which the right to self-determination in regard to treatment is insisted upon. But it is made clear that this right is limited by the patient's duties to respect his own life and health, and to have regard to his own obligations to others, including his obligation to respect the moral responsibilities of his carers.

This framework of belief about obligations no longer informs what many people understand by patient autonomy. The phenomenon of moral pluralism suggests to some of them that there is no such thing as moral knowledge (knowledge of the objective conditions of human flourishing), so that patients should be entirely free to determine what is done to them, providing doctors and nurses are willing to do it. This is the theory of a realm of unconstrained 'private choice' applied to the exercise of patient autonomy.

But the theory, as we saw, has difficulties of principle about demarcating a private realm in which choice should be unconstrained. When this supposed private realm is intended to include doctors who collaborate in the execution of patient's choices (as, for example, in euthanasia killing) it ought to be evident that what is taking place is not truly private. Doctors who kill patients profoundly shape their own characters, and the resultant characters cannot be a matter of indifference to the rest of us. Least of all could they be a matter of indifference to the dependent elderly, or a matter of indifference for the nature and quality of medical care.

This discussion of autonomy in fact returns us to the justice issues. It is clear from Michael Horan's description of his practice in the care of the debilitated elderly that he seeks to give a proper place to respect for autonomy. But it is also clear that he resolves some of the most difficult issues which arise in caring for debilitated elderly patients by reference to considerations of justice. One of the issues which exercises Horan, tube-feeding of patients with advanced dementia, has links with the topic of Joseph Boyle's paper on the American debate about artificial nutrition and hydration. Boyle identifies arguments advanced in North America for withholding tube-feeding from patients in a persistent vegetative state (PVS) which imply that a much more extensive group of patients (including those with advanced dementia) should be thought of as having worthless lives. On that view of the patients it is difficult to see what ought to prevent people from killing them. Boyle presents a defence of the view that, with certain well defined exceptions, we owe it to the majority of PVS patients to continue feeding them. While PVS patients are not a concern of Horan's paper, there is at least the appearance of a conflict between Horan and Boyle over the kind of considerations which should determine our obligations to patients who will die without tube-feeding. In a comment on their papers I seek to show how the assumptions behind Horan's approach (which is a blanket policy of withholding tube-feeding from patients with advanced senile dementia who have no prospect of recovering the ability to swallow) may be thought to be consistent with the most fundamental requirement of justice in the treatment of patients: that one should never seek intentionally to kill them. This brief discussion paper does not, however, seek to provide a justification of what I take to be the crucial assumptions underlying Horan's approach.

In my paper on *The Living Will* Report I examine the ethical framework which underpins the Report's proposals for advance patient directives which, if the directives were enforceable, would oblige doctors to withhold treatment precisely with a view to ending a patient's life. If that is a permissible objective of choice there are no sound reasons against seeking to achieve it by positive action. It is notable that this view of the permissible content of advance directives is urged upon us in the interests of patient autonomy. Patient autonomy, as I remarked earlier, is the favoured justification for the practice of euthanasia in The Netherlands. John Keown's paper reports on his extensive empirical research into that practice. It reveals what many would have said was predictable: an inability to confine the practice to *voluntary* euthanasia. The framework of 'safeguards' is revealed as providing little effective obstacle to the slide from voluntary to non-voluntary euthanasia.

The first five papers in the volume are all concerned, in one way or another, with the limits imposed by considerations of justice to the claims which can be made in the name of autonomy. The most fundamental of these considerations is that we should avoid intentionally wronging others.

Graham Mulley, Marion Hildick-Smith and Robert Stout, as experienced geriatricians, and David Hunter from his position as a health policy analyst, are concerned in the main with a different kind of justice issue: with the social provision of good quality health care for the dependent elderly both as something they need and in order to obviate any threat to their dignity.

Mulley shows that historically there has been an absence of necessary strategic planning for the long-term care of the dependent elderly. Stout brings out some of the consequent difficulties of securing fairness in the treatment of patients. He also highlights the importance of developing understanding of the distinctive health care needs of the dependent elderly. Hunter analyses the uncertainties which surround the implementation of Government policy for community care of the elderly, and the consequent risk of a policy vacuum in this area, which would have adverse effects on care of the most dependent elderly. In the absence of clear policy commitments the potential in the medium term for conflict and confusion (involving the health service and local authorities) over care of the elderly is worrying. For the long term it is clear that the fundamental policy problem which is perceived to exist is the financing of care. The one proposition of which government seems to be convinced is that the care of a growing population of the elderly cannot be maintained on the basis of public expenditure. But the prospects for securing arrangements on the basis of insurance to provide care of those who are oldest and most in need are extremely remote.

Despite the note of optimism which Hunter strikes at the end of his paper (on the basis of anticipating a growing political influence of the elderly) the fundamental picture which emerges is not one to suggest that the prospects for justice in the care of the elderly are good in our society.

There may be felt to be some irony, therefore, about providing a picture of what is required for good quality care. But Marion Hildick-Smith's delineation of those requirements simply makes clear the standards which as a community we should at least seriously seek to meet. The clearest needs she sees in the present situation are for more skilled carers, for investment in their training, and for the provision of more suitable accommodation for care.

Against the background of confusion, uncertainty and a lack of long-term commitment on the part of Government to good quality care of the dependent elderly, it is distinctly chilling to contemplate certain currents of thought which, to the degree they gain influence, can only further marginalise the dependent elderly.

Joseph Boyle examines the proposal of the influential American bio-ethicist Daniel Callahan[2] that we may fairly deny people certain forms of health care after they have completed what Callahan calls a 'natural life span'. Boyle finds the arguments for the proposal distinctly weak.

Michael Banner discusses the health care economists' device of the QALY (quality adjusted life year) for measuring the relative worth of different health care activities with a view to determining the distribution of resources. Banner begins by remarking on the insurmountable difficulties of making the kind of calculations which the idea of a QALY suggests should be possible: they stem most importantly from the fact that there is no common measure for the range of features that we count as composing the quality of life. But if one waived those fundamental objections it is clear that specific treatments for the elderly are for the most part likely to yield small returns of QALYs. Banner shows that a policy of QALY maximization is inconsistent with the requirements of justice to the dependent elderly both in respect of fairness and of need.

Michael Banner's understanding of the claim on health care provision which the dependent elderly can rightly make is one that relates that claim precisely to the dependency and fragility of their condition. Without special care their condition renders them peculiarly liable to be *extruded* from the human community. But since our claim to belong to that community rests most surely on our humanity, a fragility which threatens to marginalise the elderly demands a care for them which affirms the humanity they share with the rest of us. In my paper, 'The Aged: non-persons, human dignity and justice' I seek to show how a current of philosophical thought, which has been influential in rationalizing bad choices in other areas of medical practice, would be amenable to rationalizing bad choices in geriatric practice. It would do so precisely by proposing that numbers of the dependent elderly – those who are demented – have no serious entitlements to health care, and indeed no serious right that their lives be respected. To the degree the proposal influenced practice we would have abandoned concern for justice for the debilitated elderly and solidarity with them.

John Finnis closes the volume with an expanded version of the illuminating comments with which, as Co-Chairman, he closed the 1990 Conference. He opens with some critical observations on the 'economism' which infects too much reflection on health care policy. As he indicates, it is inherently incapable of recognising the requirements of justice. But his principal criticism is aimed at the substance and the logic of Ronald Dworkin's views on the permanently comatose. As with the subject of Joseph Boyle's first contribution to the volume, what matters for geriatric practice is the *logic* of the viewpoint under examination. Dworkin's view that the permanently comatose would be better off dead is based, as Finnis indicates, on confusing the emotionally repugnant features of certain states of extreme deprivation with a fundamental lack of human dignity in the human beings who are in those states. Finnis concludes by reflecting on the solidarity with very deprived and debilitated human beings which is required by recognition of their dignity.

It is hoped that the entire volume will aid reflection on the health care we owe to the dependent elderly. In contemplating the challenge of securing justice for them we need to keep a clear view not only of the immediate difficulties but of the social and ideological forces which threaten to undermine the character and ethos of geriatric care.

I owe debts of gratitude to friends and colleagues both for the important parts they played in relation to the original Conferences and for the help they have given in the preparation of this volume. The Conferences received moral, intellectual and financial support from the European Association of Centres of Medical Ethics and gratitude is owing to its then President, Dr Nicole Lery (Lyon), to Professor Jean-Francois Malherbe (Louvain-la-Neuve), to Professor Paul Schotsmans (Leuven), and especially to Professor Edouard Boné SJ (Brussels). Generous financial support for the Conferences was received from others, most notably Mr T. G. A. Bowles, to whom I am greatly indebted. The organization of the Conferences was largely made possible by the Deputy Director of The Linacre Centre, Mrs Agneta Sutton, and she has helpfully relieved me of some of my duties during the preparation of this volume. I am most grateful to her. The whole enterprise would not have been possible without the enthusiastic support given to it by the Governing Body of The Linacre Centre. Particular debts of gratitude are owing to its Chairman and Vice-Chairman, Professor John Utting and Professor John Finnis. They were active participants in the Conferences and unfailing sources of encouragement and advice.

It has been a pleasure to collaborate with the contributors to this volume in producing it. A number are friends of long standing and others have become friends in the course of this enterprise. Finally, I am most grateful for the exemplary patience and kind advice of Mr Peter Silver, Medical Editor at Cambridge University Press.

Luke Gormally
The Linacre Centre, August 1991.

Notes

1 The member Centres of the Association come from some dozen Western European countries. Membership is due to extend to a number of Centres in Eastern European countries.
2 Daniel Callahan. *Setting Limits. Medical Goals in an Aging Society*, New York, 1987.

2

Difficult choices in treating and feeding the debilitated elderly

MICHAEL HORAN

Introduction

In considering the topic of this chapter, I have decided to restrict myself to the problems encountered in the management of patients in hospital-based continuing care and the major assumption that underlies all my reasoning for treatment decisions in this setting is that a doctor is not always obliged to seek to prolong life when a patient is in a condition of underlying decline. Similar patients will be encountered in other settings, in which case the same assumption is relevant.

One point that is important to emphasise at the outset is that we are not dealing with a *homogeneous* group, but with a group of individuals with one thing in common; they require considerable skilled nursing care owing to severe physical disabilities, often with super-added dementia. The *common* need of such patients is *social* insofar as they are heavily dependent on others for many or all activities of daily life. Whether such a person who so wishes can be maintained at home will depend on the degree of physical and economic support that can be marshalled. The lack of willing and able family and friends or of the necessary finance to pay for the support required may remove all options other than institutional care. By way of contrast, the *medical* needs of residents of continuing care wards are enormously diverse and demanding of interventions specifically fashioned for each individual.

Despite a fairly extensive (if somewhat fragmented) literature relevant to this topic, I have elected to give a personal account derived largely from my own practice of 'Continuing Care Medicine'. However, before giving this account, it will be useful briefly to examine the context within which this type of medicine must be practised since ethical dilemmas may arise therefrom.

Demographic considerations

The term '*the greying of nations*' was introduced as a metaphor for the demographic changes that have taken place in all industrially developed countries over the course of this century. In former times, our population profile resembled a pyramid with very large numbers of young people at the base and very few old people at the apex. Our present population profile resembles more a spinning top than a pyramid with a contraction of the base and an expansion of the apex. This altered population profile is attributable to two factors: an increased life expectancy and a fall in the birth rate. Thus, our population is becoming 'top heavy' with old people. Indeed, it is interesting to note that there are more people alive in Britain today over the age of 75 than under the age of five. Even more astonishing is the fact that there are more old people alive today than have lived in the entire history of the human race.

Similar demographic changes have been recorded in all developed countries. Provided the political will is there, these rich countries should be able to deal with the economic consequences of having a large segment of the population that does not make any significant contribution to the creation of wealth. However, similar demographic trends have also been detected in developing countries (e.g. life expectancy in China is now over 70 years), usually without a significant reduction in birth rate. It seems likely that the economic consequences of increased life expectancy in such countries will become a matter of grave concern in the coming decades.

The reasons for this increase in life expectancy are imperfectly understood. The astonishing advances in medical technology seem not to have played a major part while such public health measures as clean water supplies and waste disposal as well as an improvement in nutrition and housing have contributed much. Despite the fact that the practice of medicine has contributed little to the increase in life expectancy, the aged are major consumers of health care resources. While being old is not synonymous with being diseased and disabled, old people are much more likely to suffer from disease, particularly chronic and disabling disease such as arthritis, stroke and dementia. Not only are they much more likely to have disease, it is not uncommon for several diseases to co-exist in the same individual, all of which will likely contribute to physical frailty. Furthermore, the underlying process of aging makes old people peculiarly vulnerable to the effects of not only disease but also of treatment, and serious adverse reactions to drugs account for, or contribute to, large numbers of acute admissions to hospital.

Social aspects of old age

When referring to social problems of the aged, people are usually referring to particular practical problems encountered most commonly among
old people. Poverty is probably the most pernicious of the factors predi-
sposing to 'social problems' in old age. J. K. Galbraith, the American
economist said:

People are poverty stricken when their income, even if it is adequate for survival,
falls markedly below that of the community. Then they cannot have what the
community regards as the minimum necessary for decency and they cannot wholly
escape, therefore, the judgment of the larger community that they are indecent.
They are degraded, for in the literal sense they live outside the grades or categories
which the community regards as acceptable   *(see Muir Gray, 1985).*

Those whose incomes are below the minimum necessary for subsistence
are said to be in absolute poverty. Our best estimate for the U.K. is that
about 2 million people of pensionable age live near or below the poverty
line. Poverty predisposes to poor housing, poor nutrition, lack of adequate heating and limited mobility potential. When disease and disability
are superimposed on poverty, it becomes extremely difficult for some
people to sustain an independent existence despite their desire to do so.

Planning the provision of health care

The rapid increase of an unassertive and financially compromised group
that is also a major consumer of health care resources has presented major
problems to health care planners. By and large, elderly people in the U.K.
have not made any financial provision for receiving private medical care,
and even those who have frequently find that their health care insurance is
largely geared to acute, self-limiting disorders and does not provide cover
for chronic disease and disability necessitating ongoing medical intervention. Thus, the aged are almost entirely dependent on the National Health
Service for the provision of their medical care. This leads to considerable
problems for a system that many of us know is under-funded. While it is
true that spending on health care has indeed increased in real terms, it has
not kept pace with need, let alone demand. Presently, the National Health
Service does manage to cope with the emergency workload but fails to
provide an adequate service for those conditions that are not life-
threatening. Conditions such as arthritis affecting the hip joints, must, of
necessity, be given a relatively low priority. Because so many 'orthopaedic
beds' are occupied by trauma victims, many of whom are elderly women

with hip fractures, waiting times for elective joint replacement may be as long as 18 months to 2 years. Similarly, the waiting time for cataract extraction is of comparable length and, because of financial constraints, the optimal procedure of lens implant may not be performed for those who actually get to the top of the list. Many of those waiting for hip replacement or cataract surgery live on a knife edge of coping and most geriatricians will know of patients who cannot be maintained at home because of the increasing disability attributable to the hip arthritis or visual impairment. This leads to serious conflicts for geriatricians, orthopaedic surgeons and ophthalmologists. If such a patient is advanced in the queue for restorative surgery, many more people will be pushed further down the list. If they are not advanced, some form of institutional care may be the only feasible option.

Very recently, major reforms have been taking place in both the National Health Service and in the Social Security system in Britain. It is neither appropriate nor possible for me to describe these in detail but I would like to highlight one or two areas of special relevance to my topic. Firstly, the emphasis on long-term care provision has undergone a major shift from the public sector (i.e. hospital long-term care wards) to the private sector (namely private nursing homes). Considerable amounts of public money in the form of Social Security Benefits are now being channelled into the private sector and there has been a veritable explosion in the number of private nursing homes. Supervision of the quality of care in the private sector is rudimentary to say the least. At present, the responsibility for private nursing home registration is with the local Health Authorities. While basic features such as building and fire safety and numbers of residents are carefully scrutinised, no attempt has been made to examine the nature of care provided, to ensure adequate staff training for what is a specialised branch of nursing, to require continuing education of nursing home personnel nor to determine the appropriateness of placement of individual residents. I do not mean to criticise Health Authorities for this. The law, quite simply, makes no provision to ensure such quality of care in the private sector. As a geriatrician, I see an increasing number of nursing home residents coming under my care because of acute illnesses who, in my opinion, did not require placement in a nursing home at all. It seems that the original placement was the easiest solution to a problem rather than the most appropriate solution. Often, alternatives seem not to have been considered or too readily discounted. It seems that the effect of present legislation is to return us to the situation that the British pioneers of Geriatric Medicine encountered when long-term care institutions became incorporated into the National Health Service in 1948. However, this situation will soon change as the recently enacted Griffiths proposals come into force. When people are to enter continuing care in the private sector and are financed from public funds, a multidisciplinary assessment will be made to ensure the appropriateness of placement. What is not yet clear is how these assessments will be made, by whom and what they will cost.

Attitudes to aging

The quotation from Galbraith suggests that poverty stricken old people are likely to be held in low esteem by the rest of society. In times gone by, such people would often be sent to the Workhouse. Workhouses were places to house the disabled and destitute and only the bare essentials for life were provided. The able-bodied were expected to perform work in return for this charity while the frail and disabled were simply 'warehoused' until they finally succumbed. Not surprisingly, workhouses were places to be feared. Many elderly people still remember the stigma attached to the workhouse and many Geriatrics Units are housed in former workhouses. Not surprisingly, many old people associate admission to a Geriatrics Unit with a final loss of liberty (akin to imprisonment for one who has committed no crime save to grow old) and efforts to explain otherwise are often regarded with deep suspicion – 'people only come out of such places in a coffin and I would rather die in my own home'. However, in reality, permanent hospitalisation is undertaken only when all other options prove impossible. Unfortunately, this fear of loss of liberty and self determination may predispose to the late presentation of disease in old age and a restriction of the number of therapeutic options.

Another factor that predisposes to late presentation of disease in old age is the assumption that all the changes seen in old age are due to being old and are therefore irremediable. This phenomenon is an aspect of ageism, a prejudice shared by young and old alike and sometimes by their medical attendants and other health care workers.

As a result in part of ageist beliefs and in part of social attitudes belonging to the last century, old people tend towards a rather pessimistic and sometimes fearful view of life. Before the advent of the Welfare State, many had endured extreme degrees of poverty and deprivation throughout life. What I might regard as deprivation may be as nothing compared to what they have endured in years gone by. Thus, expectations tend to be rather low. Also stemming from the time before the Welfare State is the lack of assertiveness, the unwillingness to demand their rights and the reluctance to question people in authority, so common in the aged. This makes the aged, as a group, peculiarly prone to agree to interventions they do not particularly want. It is therefore essential to take time to explain the nature of the problem and clearly to state the choices open to the patient and not simply to say 'I recommend that you undergo this or that investigation or treatment'. It is also important not to assume that the patient's assent to hospital admission automatically implies consent to any and every intervention a physician deems necessary.

The nature of ethical decision making

It should now be clear from the previous discussion that old age establishes a unique framework for the practice of medicine:

1. The aging process makes people strikingly vulnerable to the acquisition and the effects of disease, many of which are chronic and severely disabling and some, such as senile dementia, relentlessly progressive.
2. Those suffering these diseases often have a rather fatalistic view of the aetiology and prognosis of their diseases and disabilities.
3. Disease and disability in old age are likely to have profound social implications.
4. Old people tend to be unassertive and may not resist interventions that they are not convinced are in their best interests.
5. Old people are likely to have a rather different system of values than their medical attendants and other health care professionals, who are usually considerably younger. What might seem an intolerable burden to a 24-year-old House Physician might be regarded with equanimity by an 85-year-old widow, and vice versa.
6. A tendency to regard old people as a homogeneous group, 'the elderly', that is, by virtue of age alone, incapable of making sensible decisions.

In both the practice of clinical medicine and the provision of health resources, Geriatric Medicine is bristling with ethical issues and this should be obvious to anyone working with the aged. The high prevalence of severely disabling and life-threatening conditions often raises questions about how aggressively or how extensively to treat. There are two major components to any treatment decision; feasibility and desirability. Whether an intervention is feasible depends on predicting the likely outcome of the intervention. Such predictions are not easy and it should be borne in mind that while a treatment may benefit a failing organ, it will not necessarily bring about a restoration of reasonable health and may even prolong a patient's dying.

Whether a treatment is desirable raises the issue of *quality of life*, a term that has no precise, well defined meaning. Use of the term rests on a distinction between the *condition* of a human life and its *meaning and value* which involve the perception of individual worth and well-being. It must be stated unequivocally that no medical treatment can give meaning to life. The best that can be hoped for is to promote the physical function, mental alertness and emotional stability necessary for its attainment.

The financial implications of managing disease and disability in old age are immense and in the last year of life more expensive medical and social resources are consumed than in any other. Hitherto, the financial consequences of medical intervention were kept largely separate from the actual practice of medicine in the U.K. Direct financial responsibility may well be at odds with what a physician perceives as being in a patient's best interests and lead to biased decision making. It is interesting that in other circumstances such as in industry and commerce, the law requires safeguards against such *conflicts of interest*. With the present reorganisation of the National Health Service, conflicts of interest appear to be part of the fabric of the system and dilemmas hardly encountered by the medical practitioner only a few years ago are starting to arise quite often. My perception is that this reorganisation is producing a bewildering, often frustrating, health care environment in which patients' rights are easily overlooked. Physicians must make a conscious effort to fulfil their primary role as a patient's advocate and not accept the provision of sub-standard health care simply because of his or her budget responsibilities and age alone must never be permitted to become a means by which the costs of health care provision are contained.

Because ethical dilemmas are commonplace in geriatric practice, geriatricians must all be ethicists of a sort. But how do we arive at our decisions? True, we all hold our own set of moral beliefs and values, but a number of scholars looking at ethical problems in medicine in recent years have emphasised the basic importance of the following principles:

Autonomy
Beneficence
Nonmaleficence
Justice

It is important to note that an ethicist's perception of these principles may differ markedly from those of a practising clinician.

In practice, major dilemmas tend to arise only when two or more of these principles are thought to come into conflict. The principle of respect for *autonomy* or *self-determination* is given precedence over other considerations in many ethical discussions originating from the U.S.A., Western Europe and the Antipodes. In the clinical setting presently under consideration, autonomy is frequently compromised through diminished mental competence. In such circumstances it is right and proper to exercise *paternalism* – mainly motivated by the principle of justice in treatment decisions. However, one should not too readily assume lack of competence as the following example illustrates:

Mrs AW is a widow aged 86 who lives with a rather shy, unassertive, unmarried daughter. Approximately six years ago she suffered a stroke that took away her power of speech and left her with a profound weakness of the right side of her body. She is also quite deaf. She fell at home and sustained a fracture of her right hip. In line with present practice, arrangements were made to operate with a view to stabilising her broken bone by pinning the two ends together. This approach has the advantage of permitting weight bearing within a day or two of the operation, thus avoiding the possible complications of prolonged bed rest under traction (an alternative approach to treatment).

On the evening before surgery was due to take place, another daughter telephoned to say that the operation should be cancelled because she did not wish her mother to be exposed to the risks of surgery at her age. She also stated that she did not want her mother to be told that she had a broken hip because this news might cause her distress. This daughter emphasised that she would take legal action if her views were not heeded.

The following day I was asked to see the patient and was able to determine that the patient had normal comprehension, even though actually communicating with her was very difficult. I explained the nature of the problem together with the potential risks and benefits of operative treatment and of bed rest with traction. She elected for surgery and her daughter is still exploring the possibility of litigation.

Had this assertive daughter not arrived on the scene, the path to surgery would almost certainly have been followed without appropriate discussion with the patient.

The reverse of the situation just described may also be encountered when a patient refuses treatment. The family may allege neglect and assert that the patient's refusal of treatment should not have been relied upon.

Considerations of justice are already important in decisions about health care resources and their importance will increase when groups of doctors become responsible for their own budgets. I believe this will become an important source of ethical dilemmas when doctors not only function as health care providers and advocates for the needs of their patients but also as rationers of a limited budget. In this system a doctor will have to function both as counsel for the prosecution and counsel for the defence as well as being judge, jury and even executioner.

Before any particular problem can be subjected to detailed analysis, it must be ensured that sufficient information is available and that the information is accurate. Many practical dilemmas which on the face of it are ethical evaporate as detailed and accurate medical and social information is acquired. For example, in a severely confused person, decisions about fluid treatment, nutritional support or antibiotic treatment will often differ according to whether the patient had a reversible, subacute confusional state or an established, relentlessly progressive, dementing illness. Likewise, in a patient with severe psychomotor retardation, such a dementing illness may be present (which is irreversible) or there may be a severe depressive illness that might well respond to appropriate treatment. However, the quest for accurate information should not be pursued at all costs. Certain diagnostic tests carry appreciable risks, may be uncomfortable or unpleasant and constitute a scarce resource. If the result would not alter management, such investigations should not be carried out.

As well as the need for adequate information, one must also examine one's motives in arriving at a decision. Clearly, motives such as maintaining the throughput of a ward, getting rid of an extremely difficult patient or getting some sleep after a busy weekend 'on call' should play no part in clinical decision making. However, without formally examining one's motives in a particular setting, considerations such as these have a habit of intruding subconsciously. Of more relevance here are quality of life decisions in which one tries to place oneself in the patient's circumstances. You might consider that life at the age of 85 with diabetes mellitus complicated by peripheral arterial disease leading to gangrene of the toes, peripheral neuropathy resulting in diminished sensation in the feet and kidney failure would be burdensome and neglect to refer the patient to an ophthalmologist to prevent loss of vision due to diabetic eye disease. The truth might be that the individual continues to have a fulfilling life, enjoying the companionship of his wife of 60 years. It is impossible adequately to judge someone else's quality of life. Indeed, this has been emphasised in a paper by Ouslander and colleagues. They compared decisions about a group of four clinical vignettes which described medical interventions of varying risk. A low degree of correlation was found between the conclusions arrived at by mentally competent residents of an American nursing home and those of doctors, nurses, social workers and relatives. Obviously, such results are not generalisable and similar studies need to be conducted.

The motives of the family must also be considered. The 60-year-old spinster who has devoted the last ten years to looking after her dementing father may want 'everything possible to be done' because of the immense emptiness that would be left in her life, should her father die. Sometimes family members may make such requests out of a sense of guilt, having provided little support over the last few years and now it is too late to make amends. Of course, baser motives such as acquiring a patient's property or money might prompt representations not to provide life-saving treatments.

Respect for people and autonomy

The right of individuals to make independent judgments about what is and is not done to them is firmly defended in the law, especially in America. In many discussions on clinical ethics, patient autonomy is given precedence over other considerations. If a patient's right to self determination is to be properly exercised the patient needs to be well-informed about the possible options for treatment. If not well-informed a patient cannot give informed consent to treatment. In the absence of informed consent, medical intervention might be found to be battery in British law.

Informed consent implies:

1. The patient is competent
2. The patient *is* fully informed
3. The patient is not coerced

As I have previously mentioned, it is very easy to find oneself, without thinking rather than out of any conscious intention, not providing sufficient information for the patient to make a real choice. Indeed, by assuming that a patient's mere willingness to be admitted to hospital automatically implies consent, decisions about investigation and treatment may be made on behalf of a perfectly competent patient and the first the patient knows about the decision may be when the porter arrives to take him/her to the X-ray department or the nurse arrives with a new tablet or medicine. Because many older patients feel intimidated by the medical hierarchy and tend to be rather unassertive, they may reluctantly submit to such intrusions.

The issue of competence is particularly problematic in geriatric practice. In the case of apparent mild cognitive impairment, it is often difficult to determine whether the patient is not competent to make decisions or whether they are simply applying a different system of values to those of the attending medical staff. Furthermore, competence is not an all or nothing phenomenon and may vary over time. It may also vary in degree and it is quite possible not to be competent to manage financial affairs but still be able to grasp the essentials of the relative risks and benefits of some proposed surgical intervention. However, there are no precise guidelines about what constitutes competence and this is almost always left to the judgment of individual medical practitioners.

Bio-ethicists and moral philosophers have written most extensively about decisions arising within the acute care setting and in circumstances where life and death are at stake. It is in such settings that notions of autonomy and informed consent have been strongly emphasised and scant attention has been paid to decision making in the continuing care setting where Moody has argued that the informed consent standard is a dangerously limited approach to the principle of autonomy, and, further, that the ideal of autonomy itself should be understood as *a moral good, not a moral obsession*. It remains a valid and important goal for which to strive, but it is not a moral straitjacket that prohibits the exercise of paternalism in any guise. There are, in fact, circumstances where justice and/or beneficence can and should take precedence over autonomy.

The appropriate emphasis given to the requirement of informed consent in the acute care setting too often goes with a narrowly conceived view of the relationship between doctors and patients. Strict insistence on this requirement in the long-term care setting, argue McCullough and Wear, would serve to frustrate autonomy and erode quality of life, not only for the individual patients but also for other patients in the same ward.

The application of ethical principles within a long-term care setting must be anchored within the art of the possible and feasible. This setting is one where choices *are* limited. For most patients, there is no possibility of moving from a hospital long-term care ward, even if they are desperately unhappy there, and the slavish attachment to the wishes of one individual may result in infringement of the rights of another. A long-term care ward must be an ordered environment where concern is expressed for the legitimate demands of all residents. Moody has argued that in an environment where the views of many interested parties contend, where the boundaries of competence are blurred and where both the rights and the wishes of all cannot be accommodated, a new notion of *negotiated consent* needs to be employed. In this model, all interested parties are involved in consultation and negotiations are continued until a consensus is reached and a decision is possible. A final decision which the patient will accept might turn out to be the opposite of what the patient originally wanted.

We have tried to implement such a system in a limited way in the male long-term care ward for which I am responsible. In our system, all patients newly resident on the ward become the subject of a review procedure about eight weeks after admission. We have found that such reviews are extremely time consuming and can be extremely painful for some interested parties and some system of support must be available for those who suffer pain as a result. For example, one man who had diabetes that was difficult to control, who had undergone bilateral leg amputation and who was incontinent of both urine and faeces, was admitted to this ward because his wife and son were no longer able to look after him at home. Discharge home was never offered as an option to him and placement in a private nursing home could not be pursued because of the dire financial consequences for his wife. At the review meeting, he was able to express his anger and frustration about his severe medical problems and his unwilling placement on a long-stay ward. He singled out his wife as the villain of the piece and resurrected long forgotten and deeply embarrassing marital disharmonies from the past. The wife required numerous counselling sessions to work through her feelings of guilt and the patient reluctantly accepted that he had no effective choice but to remain in an environment he found deeply distressing. He rejected further attempts to permit him to work through his feelings about this decision.

The management of disturbed behaviour

On the ward to which I have just alluded, a male long-term care ward, all but three patients have severe cognitive impairment due to either the form of dementia known as Alzheimer's disease or to the dementia associated with recurrent strokes (so-called multi-infarct dementia). The natural history of Alzheimer's disease is to be relentlessly progressive over a prolonged period of time. That of multi-infarct dementia is of recurrent episodes of 'stroke'. For most of these patients, regardless of the aetiology of the dementia, the path is downhill. As a dementia progresses, aspects of the usual personality tend to become heightened. Those who were habitually loving and friendly may become more so. Those who were irritable and aggressive may also become more so. For this latter group, when remediable causes are absent and attempts at behavioural modification have failed, it is common to have to consider the use of psychotropic medication to control aggression for the protection of staff and other patients. Such drugs are very commonly associated with side effects. They may make confusion worse and quite often induce drowsiness. It is not always possible to find an appropriate treatment schedule that controls the unacceptable behaviour and yet does not induce drowsiness. Under such circumstances, protection of staff and other patients takes precedence and a treatment protocol is initiated that does not directly benefit the patient.

Life-sustaining antibiotic treatment

The discovery of antibiotics is one of the major achievements of modern medicine. They are usually effective in the treatment of infections in people of all ages but they cannot modify the underlying diseases and disabling conditions that predispose to the acquisition of the infections. Decisions about whether or not to give antibiotics eventually arise for almost all continuing care ward residents. Antibiotics are often regarded by lay people as innocuous drugs but, in fact, they may give rise to serious complications and even death. A special problem in a continuing care ward is that the widespread and frequent use of antibiotics selects strains of bacteria that are resistant to the antibiotics that are routinely available. Alternative agents tend to be either more expensive or more toxic and if these other agents are used frequently, resistance will again be a problem arising in the use of these agents as well. It is for these reasons that the use of such agents is restricted. Resistant bacteria can be created in a long term care ward and be inadvertently introduced into another place such as an intensive care unit and cause havoc. A narrow view of a doctor's duties to any individual patient under these circumstances may lead to culpable negligence since the health and lives of others who are unknown may eventually be compromised. While one should give a patient what is owed in the form of treatment from which they might significantly benefit, justice demands that others are not unfairly harmed by these actions. A doctor who works in such a setting must face up to this joint responsibility.

In a continuing care ward, about 25–30% of infections that are treated with appropriate antibiotics still prove fatal, probably because of the additional stress an infection places on one who is particularly weakened by their underlying diseases and disabilities. This observation helps in making prospective decisions about antibiotic therapy and emphasises the need for regular assessments of patients in continuing care. Those who are stable but acquire an infection as an incidental event warrant treatment while those undergoing an inexorable decline, often with a history of recurrent, recent, treated infections do not since such treatment is clearly not influencing the course of their decline, merely prolonging it. Inevitably, such decisions require value judgments about the potential outcome of treatment and the possible risks to others; these decisions should be left to those experienced in such matters i.e. the consultant in charge.

Decisions about nutritional support and fluid administration

Decisions about withholding nutritional support and/or fluids are probably the most controversial of the ethical problems we have discussed so far. The symbolic nature of nutrition and hydration is frequently an important factor in discussions about this aspect of care, and the failure to provide them, even when tubes to the stomach or intravenous procedures are needed, is of deep concern to many people. They would argue that giving food and drink is not to be considered a medical intervention. I cannot accept this and take the view that when they must be given by medical means (e.g. tubes of various sorts), the administration of food and drink does not differ fundamentally from any other category of medical intervention. It is important to note that those who are terminally ill often reduce their intake of food and fluid. When death is imminent, this can reduce nausea, vomiting, abdominal pain and lung secretions and saliva that can cause gagging and choking. This can therefore improve quality of life. Little is known about the effects when death is not imminent and some people can go on for a long time after food and fluid have been withdrawn.

In practice, the availability of complete nutrition through intravenous catheters (total parenteral nutrition) is severely limited because it requires highly specialised knowledge, is very expensive and is associated with frequent complications. For continuing care patients, feeding via a tube passed through the nose into the stomach or through the skin into the stomach (gastrostomy) are the only realistic means of providing nutrition to those who reject food by mouth. Fluids can be given by this route, by intravenous catheters and by catheters placed just under the skin. All of the possible ways of giving food and fluids have risks. For example, the insertion of tubes through the nose down to the stomach is not pleasant and often causes gagging and the patient may not properly appreciate the reason for its presence and promptly remove it. Sometimes the tube goes into the lungs and not the stomach and fluids or nutrients infused into the lungs may cause serious problems. Similarly, intravenous drips may be uncomfortable as well as being a possible site for the development of infections.

Provided a patient wishes to take food and fluids by mouth, there can be no question of withholding them on any grounds. The dilemma arises when patients reject food. Under these circumstances, it is important to make a detailed assessment of the situation. If the patient is close to death, I usually have no problem in deciding to withhold food and fluid. In other circumstances, the reason may be a positive decision of a mentally competent person, it may reflect a complicating mental disorder such as depression (which is amenable to treatment), it may reflect a problem in controlling the swallowing mechanism or it may represent a blockage in the food pathway.

When a mentally competent person makes a positive decision to reject food and fluids, this decision should be respected. If underlying depression is suspected, the help of a psychiatrist or psychogeriatrician should be enlisted, though I have not yet encountered circumstances where they have been prepared to impose treatment on such a patient against his or her wishes. If there is mechanical obstruction, it is usually possible to relieve this fairly simply by means of stretching the blockage or putting a tube through it by using a gastroscope (a sort of telescope made of flexible glass fibres). This procedure is usually well tolerated. Alternatively, a tube may be passed through the skin into the stomach, thus bypassing the blockage. Such procedures are usually justified for symptomatic relief in those for whom death is not imminent.

When a disorder of the control of swallowing is present, possible methods to alleviate the problem are more limited. In a mentally clear patient, the problem is usually caused by recurrent strokes or certain degenerative diseases of the brain. Sometimes, a speech therapist is able to suggest certain manoeuvres that lead to improvement. If these fail, the options are either some form of tube feeding, giving fluids intravenously or under the skin or no treatment at all. If the patient is competent, his views should be respected. If not, one is in the same situation as for those who are severely demented.

As dementia progresses, patients lose appreciation of their surround-ings and they may cease to recognise those close to them. Usually, by this time, such patients would not feed themselves or drink when food or drink may be placed before them. There will be times when the patient will be reluctant to swallow food or liquid placed in his mouth and attempts to promote swallowing result in inhalation, food going down the wrong way. This may precipitate an episode of choking and may even cause serious pneumonia. When such episodes become frequent, nurses become more and more reluctant to give food and drink. The issue then arises whether to provide fluid and possibly food by an artificial means. Except in situations where recovery of swallowing ability seems possible, I have a blanket policy that no artificial means should be attempted. It seems reasonable to assume that if a patient is rejecting food and drink, they are not experiencing hunger or thirst. Of course, I do not know for sure. At such times, the mouth is kept clean and moist for patient comfort and death will supervene, usually in a few days to a week or two. I have no moral dilemma in making such decisions. However, such decisions may give rise to conflicts, especially with the family. Relatives may insist on interventions that I consider futile. Such insistence may arise out of many feelings, for example love or guilt. In some circumstances, I will take time to explain the decision and the reasons why it was taken but I have not yet acquiesced in such demands. Usually, relatives accept my reasoning but occasionally they become deeply upset and angry. Very rarely they may even seek some sort of disciplinary action against me. It would be very easy to be deflected by such threats and impose an intervention that I believe would be futile (in the sense of producing no detectable benefit) and cause distress and suffering to the patient.

Acknowledgement

I am indebted to Prof. Raymond Tallis and Dr Carl Whitehouse for helpful discussions and reading the early draft of this manuscript. However, the views expressed are my own, and, for them, I accept full responsibility.

References

McCullough, L. & Wear, S. Respect for autonomy and medical paternalism reconsidered. *Theoretical Medicine*, 1985 6:295–308.
Moody, H. R. From informed consent to negotiated consent. *The Gerontologist*, 1988 28 (Suppl):64–70.
Muir Gray, J. A. Social and community aspects of aging. In: *Principles and*

Practice of Geriatric Medicine. Pathy, M. S. J. [Ed]. Wiley, Chichester. 1985 pp. 42–4.

Ouslander, J. G., Tymchuk, A. J. & Rahbar, B. Health care decisions among elderly long-term care residents and their potential proxies. *Archives of Internal Medicine*, 1989 149:1367–72.

3

The American debate about artificial nutrition and hydration

JOSEPH BOYLE

The American debate about withholding artificially provided food and water is a sprawling controversy. It includes not only strictly moral but also legal questions, and is concerned with withholding food and water provided to patients in a variety of conditions by a variety of techniques. My discussion of this controversy will, therefore, involve some simplifications. The result I hope for is a presentation of the essential contours of the moral debate, along with my own evaluation, and not a summary and critique of the details of the many arguments.

My first simplification is to focus as much as possible on the moral controversy and to avoid the strictly legal matters. Thus, although I will have something to say about recent legal decisions, it will be with a view to their moral relevance.

My second simplification is to examine just two, precisely defined and closely related kinds of human action in which the treatments withheld and the patients from whom they are withheld are specified. The treatments to be withheld in the two kinds of actions I will consider are the provision of food and water by way of a nasogastric tube or by way of a gastrostomy (a surgical procedure which provides direct access to the patient's stomach). The patients from whom these treatments are withheld in these kinds of actions are those who will live for some time in a permanently unconscious condition.

The two kinds of actions I will consider differ only in regard to whether there is prior authorization by the patient of the decision taken. In the first kind, the treatment is withheld from permanently unconscious patients on the basis of the decision maker's own judgment about what it is appropriate to provide and withhold from the patient without a prior statement by the patient concerning the decision. In the second kind, *decision makers* proceed on the basis of instructions which the patient issued while still capable of doing so.

Focusing on these two kinds of actions allows for a clear statement of the moral question which is at the center of the American debate: Supposing that all we take into account about a decision is that it is a decision to withhold either a nasogastric tube or a gastrostomy (or the use of a gastrostomy already in place) from a patient who is permanently unconscious, by decision makers who do not have prior authorization from the patient, can we judge that the decision is morally permissible or morally impermissible? Similarly, if an action is described exactly as above except that the decision makers proceed on the basis of prior instructions from the patient, can we judge that the decision is morally permissible or morally impermissible?

This way of structuring the inquiry may appear excessively abstract. I think it is not, because, as I understand the American debate, actions described in just these ways, and not all the possible variations and specifications of them, are the focus of the disagreement. Moreover, this approach highlights three kinds of morally relevant aspects of the actions in question: the condition of the patient, the nature of the treatments, and the position of the decision makers in relation to the patient's will in the matter. These are the central elements at issue in the debate.

1 The moral relevance of permanent unconsciousness

Since the discussion of the moral relevance of permanent unconsciousness remains hypothetical and dangerously speculative unless it is possible to determine that a person is permanently unconscious, I will begin with a brief summary and reflection upon the relevant medical information.

(a) The Diagnosis of persistent vegetative state

The condition of permanent and long term unconsciousness is a medical reality. At least some of the persons who are in what physicians call 'persistent vegetative state' or PVS can live for many months and even years in a condition of permanent unconsciousness.

A person is said by physicians to be in a 'vegetative state' when cognitive function is absent and only certain vegetative functions remain. Most patients in this condition can breathe and swallow spontaneously and some can chew. Most maintain a normal body temperature. Some can grimace, smile and make non-verbal sounds, and some respond to noises and movements, but not in a sustained or purposeful way. Patients in vegetative state go through cycles of sleep and wakefulness, but even while awake are incapable of any but autonomic responses and are unable to speak or otherwise purposefully interact with the environment. Such patients appear to lack all self awareness.

Vegetative state can be a transient condition, as in the case when persons awake from that kind of coma. But it can also persist. When it persists for more than a few weeks it is called persistent vegetative state or PVS. As the length of time in this condition extends, the likelihood of recovery from it decreases. Virtually no one in this condition for more than six months regains consciousness. Nevertheless, these people are not dying in the normal sense. People in persistent vegetative state can exist for years in this condition if they are fed and provided normal nursing care.[1]

The cause of the set of symptoms clinically recognized as the vegetative state is an injury or lesion of the higher parts of the brain. Apparently, the vegetative state arises when there is overwhelming damage to the cerebral hemispheres and little damage to the lower brain which controls 'vegetative' functions. Since self awareness, including the awareness of pain, depends upon the functioning of the upper brain, patients in PVS are believed to be unconscious, and to be incapable of experiencing pain.[2]

The underlying condition of the brain is not directly accessible to medical observation. In fact, there appears to be no discrete neurological condition which constitutes PVS. Rather there is a spectrum of injury and dysfunction in the cerebral hemispheres compatible with the diagnosis of PVS. Moreover, it is possible to confuse this condition with others in which the patient is not unconscious or not permanently so.[3] Consequently, the diagnosis of PVS does not by itself guarantee the soundness of the judgment that a patient is permanently comatose. However, physicians can make this judgment with confidence when the patient has been in a vegetative state for a considerable period of time and when the cause of the neurological injury, as well as the patient's age and general health, are known.[4]

I will assume, therefore, that, while it would be a mistake to suppose that a competent diagnosis of PVS is sufficient to ground a confident prognosis of long term and permanent unconscious life, it is possible for physicians confidently and responsibly to make this prognosis in some cases.

(b) How permanent unconsciousness is relevant

In those cases in which such a prognosis is made, the question of the moral significance of the patient's condition is pointed. It is clear enough why a question arises here: a person who is permanently unconscious can never again experience anything or do anything. This means that the good which care givers can provide for the permanently unconscious is necessarily limited in its objectives. The most we can do for people in this condition is to prolong their lives and treat them with care and respect. Since our efforts can have so little good effect, all agree that it is necessary to face the question about when those efforts should be limited, and virtually all agree that those limits are reached far more quickly than in the case of patients with a better prognosis.

Many who have considered the matter of limiting treatment to the permanently unconscious regard the patient's condition as one among a set of factors which need to be taken into account. But some hold that the competent prognosis of this condition is by itself sufficient to justify the radical limitation of treatment involved in withholding food and water provided by way of a nasogastric tube or gastrostomy. They argue that, since virtually all of what people value in life involves experience and action, the life of the permanently unconscious is not simply deprived like that of anyone who is seriously and chronically ill but completely lacks value.

This perception that the lives of permanently unconscious people lack value has been articulated in two different ways – as the thesis that these people are already, in the relevant sense, dead, and as the thesis that these people cannot benefit from continued life. Before considering these two theses, it is important to note two aspects of the general idea that the lives of permanently unconscious persons lack value.

First, since the condition of permanent unconsciousness is morally relevant because it is an incapacity for experience and action, the nonarbitrary application of the general idea cannot be limited only to the permanently unconscious. Anyone who is permanently incapable of experience and action is, by virtue of the condition causing this incapacity, living a life devoid of value. Thus, life sustaining treatment should be withheld from many who are demented, but not unconscious, such as advanced Alzheimer's patients, from many retarded persons, and perhaps from people in other groups as well. Many people in these categories surely cannot act in any adequate human way, and, although many are capable of some kinds of experience, it is unclear why many of these experiences should be any more valuable than the complete lack of experience of the unconscious. Indeed, many of the people in these categories are utterly miserable; their experiences seem to be largely negative. Surely a view which links the value of a human life to its possessor's capacity for experience cannot mean to endorse just any experience as valuable.

Secondly, the reliance upon the condition of permanent unconsciousness as the sole decisive factor in decisions to withhold food and water has nothing specifically to do with these treatments. It provides an all purpose justification for withholding any treatment which sustains life, and perhaps for withholding other forms of care, and perhaps for killing these patients.

Since these implications are far reaching, acceptance of the idea that the condition of permanent unconsciousness by itself is sufficient to settle the matter is not as appealing as might at first appear. Thus, it would be reasonable to accept it, rather than the weaker view that this condition is one factor among others to be considered, only if it is supported by very powerful considerations. In fact, the arguments for the alternate versions of this view (viz. that the permanently unconscious are dead or, if not dead, cannot be benefited) are not compelling, which perhaps explains why the American debate appears to proceed largely on the weaker view.

(c) Are the permanently unconscious dead?

The first articulation of the idea that the lives of the permanently unconscious are without value is the thesis that permanently unconscious patients have in the humanly significant sense already died. In other words, it is the claim that the death of a human person occurs not at the end of the biological life of the organism, but when the higher brain functions associated with consciousness have permanently ceased. On this view, the permanently unconscious human is a living human organism, but no longer a person.[5]

This simple but extreme view of the significance of the condition of permanent unconsciousness implies that the permanently unconscious are to be treated in much the same way as we treat human cadavers; they are no longer persons who could have rights and interests which need to be considered in these decisions.

Aside from the practical difficulties of implementing so radical a redefinition of death and of the human person, this view is open to serious philosophical objections. First, it is deeply counter-intuitive: it justifies not only withholding food and water from these individuals but also killing them and making any sort of use of them whatsoever that would be appropriate in using human cadavers. Secondly, it appears to settle important ethical questions by simply redefining terms. Unless there are compelling reasons for thinking that being a living organism of the human kind is not sufficient for being a person, such a redefinition of the notion of person is nothing more than question begging stipulation. The arguments in favor of this sort of separation of the idea of a human person from that of a living human organism are notoriously unpersuasive. Thirdly, this separation implies a dubious understanding of the human person as two things – a person whose existence depends upon the working of the upper brain, and the (rest of the) human organism.[6]

(d) Does continued existence benefit the permanently unconscious?

The second way of articulating the idea that the lives of the permanently unconscious lack value is the view that they can no longer be benefited, either generally or at least by actions which prolong their lives. It seems to me that either the general or the specific version of this view underlies much of the thinking of those who favor withholding food and water from the permanently unconscious, even on the part of those who do not explicitly endorse the sufficiency of the patient's condition for justifying the withholding of the food and water. Thus, for example, even some Catholic theologians of a fairly traditional stripe appear to hold that since the permanently unconscious are no longer capable of pursuing the spiritual ends of life, any actions taken to prolong their lives are simply pointless. They serve no purpose whatsoever.[7]

The most straightforward argument for the general view that the permanently unconscious cannot be benefited has as its key premise the claim that a person's capacity to experience a benefit is a necessary condition for that person's receiving the benefit. A putative benefit which could never be experienced as a benefit by the intended beneficiary is thus not a genuine benefit.

But this claim about the nature of a benefit cannot be sustained. For it surely is possible to harm someone without their ever knowing about it. A slander may deny the person slandered some opportunities and thus harm that person even if he or she never discovers the slander. But if harms of this kind are possible then so are benefits: if one refrains from slander and thus does not deny the relevant opportunities, it would surely seem that one benefits the peson one does not slander whether or not the person ever finds out. This seems to hold in the case of the permanently unconscious: one can surely harm them, for example, by making them spectacles or by treating them like experimental animals. So, it would seem, one can benefit such persons, at least by taking steps to safeguard them from such abusive actions.

The more specific view that actions undertaken solely to prolong the lives of the permanently unconscious do not benefit them avoids controversial claims about the nature of benefits and harms. It need only involve a claim about the specific character of the benefit of continued life for those who are permanently unconscious. The essential claim seems to be that the value of continued life for a peson is contingent upon that person's capacity to do and/or experience some things.

The simplest way to understand this claim is as the proposition that human life itself is only instrumentally good; perhaps, however, the claim could be that life is inherently good but only within the larger context of the possibility of the conscious and active pursuit of other worthwhile goals.

The purely instrumental account of the value of human life surely cannot be correct. For a human person is a living organism; a person's life is himself or herself, not a thing distinct from the person which can be possessed and used as an instrument.[8]

However, the account of human life as good only contextually (though not merely instrumentally) has considerable intuitive appeal. Most of the goods human beings have reason to seek would lack appeal except within the context of the wider spectrum of activities and experiences which, taken together, make up a person's life. Moreover, the life of a permanently unconscious person is, even in terms of the immediately relevant goods of life and health, very deprived. The permanently unconscious person, although not dying, is very ill and deprived indeed. We all want more than that for ourselves and anyone we care about.

However, this view collapses into the more general view according to which the experience of benefits is a necessary condition for their existence. For according to this contextual view, any benefit which the recipient never experienced would not be a part of the good life he or she would have reason to create.

Moreover, this view that human life is good only in a relational context in which other goods can be realized is not the only way to account for the facts about human striving after basic goods. For they are compatible with the view that human life, even in the deprived condition of permanent unconsciousness, is inherently good. For it does not follow from the fact that people seek particular goods such as knowledge, excellence in work and play, friendship, and even life and health themselves as parts of a complete and fulfilling life that these goods are not inherently desirable.

On the face of it a person's life is good because these irreducible components are inherently good and not the other way round. Similarly, the fact that a good can be realized only in a limited and partial way does not generally imply that such realizations are not good at all. Partial realizations of purely instrumental goods can, of course, fail to be even marginally good, but even the very partial and limited realizations of the goods in which people find fulfillment remain instantiations of those goods, for example, the halting efforts to understand by the retarded, or the efforts to maintain health on the part of the elderly infirm.[9]

In short, the attempts to show that continued existence is not a benefit for the permanently unconscious fail. Either they proceed from a disputable theory about the nature of benefits and harms which is open to counter-examples or they accept an indefensible form of dualism. Moreover, these attempts have some of the counter-intuitive implications of the view that the permanently unconscious are no longer persons. For if the continued life of a permanently comatose person is not a benefit, ending that life cannot be a harm to that person. Thus, the prohibition against killing such people cannot be based on any interest or right of theirs. Furthermore, if the reason why continued life is not a benefit is that life has only instrumental or contextual value, then there seems to be no ground for valuing the lives of such persons. Regarding them as persons seems deprived of all practical significance.

II The moral relevance of the treatments

The upshot of the argument of the last section is that the permanently unconscious condition of the patient is not by itself sufficient ground for withholding food and water. This factor is one consideration among several necessary for arriving at a justified decision on this matter. Most of the other relevant considerations are related to the character of the treatment by which food and water are provided to these patients.

(a) Withholding food and water and intentional killing

Much of the debate about withholding food and water from the permanently unconscious centers on the question of whether this action is murder or otherwise wrongful killing of the patient. Most of those who oppose such actions do so because they regard them as murder. Much of the argument of those who favor such actions is an effort to rebut this charge.

The reasoning of those who regard this kind of action as murderous depends upon two considerations: the causality of the death and the intentions involved in the decision.

The argument from causality is that withholding food and water leads quickly and inevitably to death. The permanently unconscious from whom food and water are withheld die of starvation and dehydration, not from their underlying brain malfunction. What the brain malfunction causes is not the person's death, but his or her need to be fed and hydrated.[10]

It seems to me that, in spite of the difficulties surrounding the concept of causality, the factual observation underlying this argument is correct. For those who decide to withhold food and water do not initiate a causal chain that will lead to death, but refuse to do what will prevent death in circumstances in which there is a causal chain that will bring about death. I see no reason why the removal of what prevents death should not be considered a kind of cause. Aquinas, for example, regarded as a '*per accidens* cause' any factor which removes what prevents the occurrence of an effect.[11]

The causality of death is not, however, sufficient for the judgment that withholding food and water is murder. For the withholding of other kinds of treatment leads to death as quickly and surely as withholding food and water, and withholding these kinds of treatments is surely permissible in some cases, for example, the removal of a respirator from one who cannot breathe without it. Moreover, there are cases of withholding food and water which, while causally identical to withholding food and water from patients in PVS, are intuitively as justifiable as turning off a respirator which is essential for life, for example, when food and water is given to some and denied to others because of scarcity, or when a conscious patient refuses food and water because of disagreeable features of the methods of feeding and hydrating.

These examples suggest that intention is the crucial factor in determining that the decision to withhold food and water is murderous. For even if the carrying out of the decision to withhold food and water causes death, the decision can be morally acceptable if death is not intended. Moreover, if the patient's death is intended – if its occurrence is the reason why the decision is taken – then the decision is murderous. For intentional killing of the innocent is surely the core of the idea of murder.[12]

Furthermore, the decision to withhold food and water is an intentional action in the relevant sense, even though it is a decision not to do something. Like other decisions, decisions not to do things are rational human actions in which certain outcomes are not simply expected and welcomed or regretted but sought and intended. Thus, not surprisingly, virtually all legal systems regard homicide by omission as a possibility.

People often seek a certain outcome by choosing not to do something. Furthermore, the fact that they would not choose some other, perhaps more effective, means to realize that outcome does not imply that they do not intend it. Thus, the fact that those who decide to withhold food and water are unwilling to take initiatives to kill the patient is not evidence that they do not intend death. There may be other good reasons, perhaps of a psychological or legal kind, which rule out more active steps to achieve their objective.

The public record concerning the best known of the American cases strongly suggests that the intentions of the decision makers in at least some of them has included the intent to end the patient's life.[13] Daniel Callahan's explanation for the renewed interest in the question of withholding food and water suggests that this intention is widespread in these decisions: 'A denial of nutrition may, in the long run, be the only way to make certain that a large number of biologically tenacious patients actually die.'[14]

The combination of the actual statements of decision makers, the apparent motivations behind the social movement towards withholding food and water, and reflection upon the intentions people might have for withholding food and water starkly raise the question of whether it is possible to make this decision without intending the patient's death.[15]

Serious reflection on the moral issue of withholding food and water from those in PVS surely requires that this question be faced squarely. But it would be a mistake to think that the answer to it must in every case be that withholding food and water is intentional killing. For there are surely benefits which might be sought by a decision to withhold food and water which do not include the patient's death – decisions in which the patient's death is not intended but accepted as a side effect of a decision taken for other reasons. This possibility does not presuppose the false view of intention as a purely mental volition, resolve or speech one makes to oneself. For although intentions are one's practical interest in the benefits to be achieved by what one chooses to do, their character is frequently not revealed by the behavior which carries out choices, and sometimes is not revealed by the choice itself, particularly when it is a choice not to do something.

(b) Is providing food and water medical treatment or normal care?

One of the major strands in the American debate has been a controversy about whether providing food and water by way of a nasogastric tube or gastrostomy should be classified as medical treatment or as normal human care of the kind provided by family members or nurses. This controversy is closely related to the disagreement about whether withholding food and water is wrongful killing. Those who hold that providing food and water in these ways is medical treatment do so as part of an argument that, like other medical treatments, it can be withheld for a variety of reasons without any presumption of wrongdoing. Those who classify these ways of providing food and water as normal human caring do so as part of an argument that withholding these treatments is either wrongful killing or wrongful refusal to care for the patient.[16]

It seems to me that at one level this debate is simply verbal. The facts are clear enough: gastrostomies are surgical operations of a fairly simple kind, and once established need no special expertise to maintain and use. Nasogastric tubes require some expertise to insert and some trained nursing care to maintain. Neither involves the use of high technology and sophisticated equipment.

The moral significance of these facts is not altogether clear. For classification of a procedure as medical does not by itself settle whether or not it is morally required, and classification as normal caring does not imply that refusal of the procedure is impermissible. Of course, the grounds for refusal of a procedure become more stringent to the extent that the procedure is part of the care we feel obliged to provide to any dependent. Thus, those who argue that withholding these ways of providing food and water is refusing normal human care raise a further question about these decisions: are they an unfair refusal of a kind of care all humans deserve?

(c) The symbolic significance of feeding and hydrating

Another strand within the American debate has been the discussion of the symbolic significance of feeding and providing water to people. Eating and drinking are elemental human activities and are often part of human interactions in which human solidarity and friendship are expressed and maintained. Thus, refusal to give a thirsty person water or a hungry person necessary food is harmful not only to life and health but to human community. Therefore, the withholding of food and water from the permanently unconscious may have a significance for care givers and the entire community which goes beyond the fact that it causes the death of the unconscious patient.[17] The objection to this line of reasoning is that in the context food and water are not provided in ways which have their normal human meaning and the recipients are not capable of the human responses which make the offer of food and drink so humanly important.[18]

I believe that underlying the concern about the symbolic significance of food and drink there is a vital moral consideration whose significance is not merely symbolic. For in providing food and drink to the permanently comatose we do what we can to help them and to remain in solidarity with them. True, the permanently unconscious patient cannot, in this world at least, ever experience the results of this human concern. But it does not follow that there is no benefit for the unconscious person. The bonds between persons which constitute human solidarity are not merely psychological, but are moral realities constituted by the choices to promote and share the goods of one's friends. Those who are unconscious are treated precisely to show respect for their essential humanity and to avoid inflicting harms which would wrong them. If, as I argued above, we are in no position to deny that continuing the life of a permanently unconscious person is a benefit to that person, we are in no better position to deny that the bonds of friendship established in this effort are really beneficial to the person helped.[19]

(d) Does providing food and water harm the patient?

Maintaining solidarity with the permanently unconscious is a good thing only if what we do for them is not harmful to them. But the normal harms to a patient do not seem to apply here because of the patient's unconscious condition: the perceived indignity of being manipulated and subjected to invasive procedures, the limitations on mobility, the constraints on doing other things, the pain of one's condition and its treatment, and so on are not harms which can afflict a permanently unconscious person. Similarly, it is hard to believe that the continued life of such a person could itself be a harm to that person.

Of course, it is possible to harm such a person: surely abusive or exploitative use of the person does that. In some cases the treatments by which food and water are provided might also harm the patient, for example, when a nasogastric tube causes infection or the patient cannot tolerate food provided by a gastrostomy. These possible harms of feeding and hydrating some permanently unconscious patients have not, however, been proposed seriously as grounds for withdrawing these treatments.

But the common contention that artificially providing food and water is harmful because it is degrading and dehumanizing seems to me without foundation.[20] For the person is not being used for alien purposes but respected and helped in the only way care givers are able.

(e) Does providing food and water impose unreasonable burdens on others?

Although providing food and water artificially is not generally a plausible harm to the patient, it can impose burdens on others. Of course, the continued life of such a person imposes certain burdens, particularly on family members. The ongoing sadness and disruption of life are very serious indeed for many families. But these burdens of the person's remaining alive are removed only by the death of the person, and so, if the decision to withhold treatment is taken to remove these burdens, it includes the intention of the patient's death.

Still, there is another kind of burden involved. The treatment of permanently unconscious patients involves costs, and the resources used to maintain them can surely be used for other worthwhile purposes. Indeed, one can easily think of situations in which families had to bear the entire costs of maintaining permanently unconscious relatives and simply could not afford to do so. Clearly, in cases like these the choice to withhold food and water would not be wrongful killing and might be morally required. However, this has not been the predicament of families of PVS patients in the United States, where most of the costs have been carried by welfare agencies.

In this context it is necessary to consider what the costs actually are. Relatively little has been said about this in the published literature. The facts seem to be that while the overall costs of taking care of the permanently unconscious over a period of time are very significant, the costs of providing food and water by a nasogastric tube or gastrostomy are not significant, either as a portion of the overall costs of care for these patients or in relation to health care costs generally.[21] It seems inescapable, therefore, that if avoiding the costs of treatment is the ground for the decision to withhold food and water, then it is the overall set of burdens involved in caring for the patient, not any specific costs of providing food and water, which the decision makers want to avoid.

It follows that the decision to withhold food and water is a decision to refuse care for the patient, and that is abandoning the patient. Sometimes, particularly in exigent circumstances, it is permissible to abandon people. But it seems that outside such conditions, as exist perhaps in crisis situations or, more routinely, in the lives of hunter–gatherer peoples living in hostile environments, abandonment cannot be justified.

The idea that health care professionals should always care for their patients, even when curing them is impossible, is an application of a general moral truth about human relationships. We should not turn our backs on fellow humans in need, even when we morally or physically cannot do much to help them. Thus, in institutionally less complex societies than our own, decent people would care for their debilitated family members as their circumstances permitted. Hardly ever would they simply abandon them to die.[22]

The fact that most of the permanently unconscious are not at home but in expensive medical facilities both highlights and raises the costs involved, and obscures the reality of abandonment. Perhaps the costs of maintaining these people in these institutions are too high, but surely there are ways to deal with this problem other than by simply abandoning them, or making sure that they starve to death so that they will not have to be wheeled out into the street.

III The moral relevance of the patient's prior authorization

In the first two sections of this paper I have been assuming that the human action in question is the act of withholding the food and hydration provided by nasogastric tube or gastrostomy from a permanently unconscious person by decision makers who lack prior authorization from the patient. It remains to consider the second of the kinds of acts I delineated there: the same decision except that the decision makers are operating on the basis of a clear prior authorization by the patient.

This difference in acts has played a significant role in the American debate, as the recent US Supreme Court decision in the Cruzan case makes clear. The Court sustained the ruling of a lower appellate court which overturned the decision of a trial court which had allowed the parents of Nancy Cruzan, a PVS patient who was clearly permanently unconscious, to withhold food and water provided by a gastrostomy. The lower court overturned the trial court's decision because Cruzan's statements about wanting to be refused such treatments if ever permanently unconscious did not meet the strict evidentiary requirements set by Missouri statute. The Supreme Court ruled that Missouri's evidentiary

requirements were compatible with the Constitution, and so strongly
suggested that had those requirements been met, the decision to withhold
the food and water from Ms Cruzan would have been legally acceptable.[23]

The moral question, of course, is whether the distinction underlying the
Court's decision – between decisions made by others with and those made
without the patient's prior authorization – makes any essential moral
difference. The moral significance of prior patient authorization depends
upon the moral significance attributed to individual autonomy.

The exercise of a competent person's autonomy in decisions concerning
the person's health care is widely accepted as a person's right: the right to
refuse treatment. This right is understood to protect discretion concerning life saving and extending treatments. In the United States that
right has been extended in recent years through such devices as living wills
and legislation allowing for the use of durable power of attorney which
allow a person to determine while still competent what treatments he or
she will accept after becoming incompetent.[24]

On the face of it this legal arrangement settles only the legal and social
question of whose decision is to be determinative in matters involving the
health care of the noncompetent. It does not address the question of what
sort of moral considerations the decision makers should address.

These distinct issues are often confused, particularly by those who
regard the exercise of personal autonomy as itself a great value, and by
those who collapse moral problems into legal problems. Thus, many
people seem to believe that a patient's decision about his or her health
care is morally justified just because it is an exercise of the patient's will.
This sort of voluntaristic subjectivism seems plainly false, whatever its
appeal in popular ethical discussion: the simple fact that a person wants
something or decides on something has no tendency to make it right.

If the patient's prior directives are not to be regarded as important
simply because they express his or her desires, it might appear that they
have no relevance in assessing the moral character of a decision to
withhold food and water. Indeed, according to many of the positions
surveyed in the earlier sections of this paper, this circumstance of the
decision is of little practical importance. For example, those who regard
the condition of the patient as by itself decisive grounds for withholding
food and water should regard the presence or absence of prior authorization as being no more than marginally important: whatever the patient
may have said about the matter, his or her life lacks value. Similarly, if
one regards the causality of death in these cases as decisive evidence that
withholding the food and water is morally prohibited killing, then the

moral difference between the two acts is like that between murder and suicide. Likewise, if one believes that withholding food and water necessarily involves the intention of death.

On the other hand, if, as I believe, the decision to withhold food and water is not necessarily murderous, then the difference between the two actions can mark the distinction between kinds of acts that are permissible and kinds that are impermissible.

I argued above that the decision to withhold food and water to avoid the costs of caring for the unconscious patient is a form of abandonment of the patient which can be justified only in the most severe and pressing of human circumstances. But suppose the patient himself or herself decides, while still competent, that those costs should be avoided so that the resources used to care for him or her could be used for some other good purpose. Such a decision is surely possible: if others can decide, even wrongly, to avoid the costs of a treatment, a person can surely make this choice concerning his or her own treatment. Thus, a person can issue a directive to the effect that he or she does not want to be fed and hydrated after becoming permanently unconscious without a suicidal intention, and, I think, without any other wrongful willing.

Those who act in accordance with such a directive are surely not acting murderously, nor are they assisting in suicide. But more importantly, they do not seem to be involved in morally objectionable abandonment of the patient. Rather, they are accepting the patient's act of generosity. The impact on the human good of solidarity is thus altogether different than if they had decided on their own to abandon the patient. As in many actions where the goods of human friendship and community are at stake, it makes a significant difference who makes the decision.[25]

I conclude, therefore, that prior authorization by the patient can cause an action which would be wrong for people to take on their own initiative to be morally good.

Still, it is plainly possible that a person issue an advance directive with suicidal intent, and that care givers know this. Even here their choice to act in accord with the directive need not involve the intention to end the person's life, but only the intention to honor the person's established right to refuse treatment. Nevertheless, the choice of decision makers to honor the patient's right to refuse treatment does provide assistance for his or her suicidal project. It seems to me that this is a case of what Catholic moralists call material cooperation. Thus, unless strictly bound by legalities or other pressing reasons, care givers should not cooperate in carrying out the patient's directive.

Notes

1 See Fred Plum, M.D., Medically altered states of consciousness, in Russell Smith, editor, *Critical Issues in Contemporary Health Care* (The Pope John Center: Braintree, MA, 1989), p. 48. This presentation by one of the recognized experts in neurology provides a useful introduction to the medical issues for laymen. See also Ronald Cranford, The persistent vegetative state: the medical reality (getting the facts straight), *Hastings Center Report* 18.1 (February/March 1988), 27–32; President's Commission for the Study of Ethical Problems in Medicine and Biomedical and Behavioral Research, *Deciding to Forego Life-Sustaining Treatment* (Washington, D.C.: U.S. Government Printing Office, 1983), pp. 174–81.

2 See Council on Scientific Affairs and Council on Ethical and Judicial Affairs (of the American Medical Association), Persistent vegetative state and the decision to withhold or withdraw life support, *Journal of the American Medical Association* 263 (1990), 428. See also Plum, *op. cit.*, pp. 57–8. Some medical disagreement about the possibility that patients in vegetative state can experience pain has recently been reported in the popular press; see *The Globe and Mail* (Canada), Vegetative patients may sense pain, July 13, 1990, p. 6.

3 The primary difficulty is in distinguishing people in 'locked in syndrome' who are conscious but unable to communicate from those in PVS; see Plum, *op. cit.*, pp. 49, 57–8; Council on Scientific Affairs, *loc. cit.* It is also worth noting that there have recently been reports of a person being revived from PVS after eight years by the use of tranquilizers; see *The Patriot Ledger* (Boston), March 28, 1990, p. 2 and March 29, 1990, p. 2. See also Recovery from persistent vegetative state?: the case of Carrie Coons, *Hastings Center Report* 19.4 (July/August 1989), 14–15.

4 The interpretation of the medical literature in this and the preceding paragraphs owes much to discussions with Paul Ranalli, M.D., Toronto.

5 The standard version of this view is that of Robert Veatch, *Death, Dying and the Biological Revolution: Our Last Quest for Responsibility* (New Haven and London: Yale University Press, 1976), pp. 25–76. Daniel Wickler, Not dead, not dying? ethical categories and persistent vegetative state, *Hastings Center Report* 18.1 (February/March 1988), 41–7 argues that patients in persistent vegetative state should be declared dead.

6 For a detailed philosophical critique of Veatch's proposal see, Germain Grisez and Joseph M. Boyle Jr., *Life and Death with Liberty and Justice: A Contribution to the Euthanasia Debate* (Notre Dame and London: University of Notre Dame Press, 1979), pp. 71–8; for a critique of the dualism involved in redefinitions of death, see pp. 70–1, and more generally pp. 372–80. Difficulties of the kind Grisez and I raised perhaps explain why the idea of 'neocortical death,' although present in the discussion since the debate about the Quinlan case in the 1970s, has had so little influence in the legal decisions, and has appeared so infrequently in the more recent ethical discussions.

7 See Kevin O'Rourke, O.P., The A. M. A. statement on tube feeding: an ethical analysis, *America*, November 22, 1986, 322; Evolution of church teaching on prolonging life, *Health Progress* (January–February, 1988), 8, 29–35, especiaslly 32–3.

8 Those who deny this seeming datum must embrace a form of the dualism criticized above; see note 6. For an elaboration of the implication of dualism

by any view which regards human life as only instrumentally valuable see John Finnis, Joseph Boyle and Germain Grisez, *Nuclear Deterrence, Morality and Realism* (Oxford: Oxford University Press, 1987), pp. 307–9.

9 See Finnis, Grisez and Boyle, *op. cit.*, pp. 305–6 for a development of this argument.

10 Parts of the argument sketched here play a role in much of the reasoning of those who reject the withholding of food and water; see, for example, Patrick Derr, Why food and fluids can never be denied, *The Hastings Center Report* 16.1 (February, 1986) 28 30. The discussion of causality also emerges in the legal cases for obvious reasons. However, the most common consideration of causality is by those who argue that the decision to withhold food and water is not the cause of death. The idea, maintained by O'Rourke and others, that the patient's underlying pathology, and not the decision to withhold the food and water, causes death seems to me either plainly false or the result of an arbitrary stipulation about what a cause is.

11 See *Summa Theologiae*, First part of the Second Part, Question 76, article 1. For a useful untangling of confusions on this subject see Dan Brock, Forgoing life-sustaining food and water: is it killing? in Joanne Lynn, editor, *By No Extraordinary Means: The Choice to Forgo Life-Sustaining Food and Water* (Bloomington and Indianapolis: Indiana University Press, 1986), pp. 126–9.

12 See The Linacre Centre, *Euthanasia and Clinical Practice: Report of a Working Party* (The Linacre Centre: London, 1984), pp. 24–36; for a philosophical argument for the conclusion that intentionally killing the innocent is always wrong see Finnis, Boyle and Grisez, *op. cit.*, pp. 297–319.

13 Most of the public statements of people involved as decision makers in these cases are ambiguous. This is so because many of them have been made in the context of legal proceedings which have involved questions about the patient's known or supposed wishes as well as other moral considerations such as the balance of benefits and burdens. Still, in some cases it is difficult to interpret the decision except as involving the intention of the patient's death. In the Brophy case, for example, Brophy's own statements while competent seem to suggest that his conditional intentions in the matter were for death, and the judge in the initial trial found that the purpose of withholding nutrition from Mr Brophy was 'to terminate his life' rather than spare him pain or discomfort; see George Annas, Do feeding tubes have more rights than patients? *The Hastings Center Report* 16.1 (February, 1986), 26 7. A summary of the final decision reports it as ruling that 'Mr. Brophy's family could have the feeding tube disconnected so that he could die.' Pat Milmoe McCarrick, Withholding or withdrawing nutrition or hydration, *Scope Note 7* (Washington D.C.: National Reference Center for Bioethics Literature, 1986, revised), 5.

14 Daniel Callahan, On feeding the dying, *The Hastings Center Report* 13.5 (October 1983), 22.

15 See Gilbert Meilander, On removing food and water: against the stream, *The Hastings Center Report* 14.6 (December 1984), 11–13 for a compelling argument for the presumption that withholding food and water involves the intention to end the patient's life. Meilander recognizes that this cannot be more than a presumption; see 13.

16 See Meilander, *op. cit.*; Patrick Derr, Nutrition and hydration: Brophy and Jobes from a historical perspective, *Issues in Law and Medicine* 2.1 (1986),

33–6. This issue has played a role in a number of the famous legal decisions and dissents.

17 See Callahan, *loc. cit.*

18 See Joanne Lynn and James Childress, Must patients always be given food and water?, *The Hastings Center Report* 13.5 (October 1983), 20–1; Ruth Casper O. P., Food and water: symbol and reality, *Health Progress* (May 1988), 54–8.

19 See Germain Grisez, Should nutrition and hydration be provided to permanently comatose and other mentally disabled persons? *Linacre Quarterly*, 57.2 (May, 1990), 38–9.

20 This is an extremely widespread belief. See Justice William Brennan, Supreme Court of the United States, Cruzan v. Director Missouri Dept. of Health, June 25, 1990, dissenting opinion at 11; for a recent variation see Lawrence J. Schneiderman, Exile and PVS, *The Hastings Center Report* 20.3 (May/June 1990), 5.

21 See Lynn and Childress, *op. cit.*, 17–18; the only description of the specific costs of feeding of which I am aware is by James Bopp, Choosing death for Nancy Cruzan, *The Hastings Center Report* 20.1 (January/February 1990), 43: 'In Nancy's case, the cost of her food is only $7.80 per day, which is only 2.6 per cent of the total cost of her care, and which is being borne entirely by the state of Missouri.' His source is a personal communication from the Administrator of the Missouri Rehabilitation Center. Virtually all of the discussions of the costs involved in these cases have focused on the overall costs of caring for these patients; see, for example, Cranford, *op. cit.*, 31–2.

22 Concern about wrongful abandonment has not so far played a major role in the American debate. It was introduced into the discussion by William E. May, *et al.*, Feeding and hydrating the permanently unconscious and other vulnerable persons, *Issues in Law and Medicine* 3.3 (Winter 1987), 203–7. This line of argument has been developed in my, Artificial provision of nutrition and hydration: does the benefit outweigh the burden in the artificial provision of nutrition and hyrdration? An affirmative answer, in Smith, editor, *op. cit.*, pp. 60–9, and by Grisez, *op. cit.*, 30–43.

23 See Supreme Court of the United States, Cruzan v. Director, Missouri Dept. of Health, decided June 25, 1990. The majority opinion was written by Chief Justice Rehnquist. Justice Scalia, in a concurring opinion, argues that following Ms Cruzan's stated wishes would be assisting in suicide, and that the state rightly restricts suicide, so he apparently would not accept the suggestion of the majority opinion that had her statements met the evidentiary requirements set by Missouri statute, withholding feeding by the gastrostomy would be legally acceptable.

24 For a discussion of the right to refuse treatment and living wills see Grisez and Boyle, *op. cit.*, pp. 86–120.

25 On this I am indebted to Grisez, *op. cit.*, 33–4.

4

Reflections on Horan and Boyle

LUKE GORMALLY

Michael Horan's paper directly reflects his clinical practice in the continuing care setting with patients who, as he says, will have suffered a dramatic loss of independence in moving from home to the geriatric unit. There are very strong reasons, therefore, for seeking to mitigate that loss by encouraging the exercise of self-determination wherever it can be appropriately exercised. Horan shows himself anxious to respect the right to self-determination of the elderly where there is the required capacity to exercise that right and where what the patient desires does not involve injustice to others.

The distinction between what a patient wants and what is required in justice in the treatment of a patient is clearly important in determining the limits of autonomy in concrete situations. When Horan comes to focus in the final part of his paper on three difficult types of decision which from time to time have to be made in the care of the debilitated elderly, it is clear that his practice is in fact governed by considerations of justice.

(1) Psychotropic medication, in dosages which cause drowsiness or induce confusion, may be required in the management of disturbed behaviour in order to avoid foreseeable harm to staff on whom the care of the patients depends. To fail to protect staff, however, would be *unfair* to them, as well as producing conditions which were not in the interests of the patients.

(2) The use of life-sustaining antibiotic treatment must be selective given the danger of creating resistant bacteria which may be introduced to other parts of a hospital (such as the intensive care unit). Underlying this view of the geriatrician's duty is, first, the assumption Horan states at the beginning of his paper: that a doctor has no overriding duty to seek to prolong a patient's life when the patient is irreversibly declining. Further, he believes that when one cannot be confident about achieving significant

47

benefit for patients with antibiotic treatment, *fairness* requires that one does not undermine the therapeutic value of that treatment for patients who would otherwise benefit from it.

(3) Finally, Horan says he has a blanket policy of not providing food and fluids through a nasogastric tube or gastrostomy to patients with advanced dementia who are repeatedly failing or refusing to swallow and who are unlikely to recover their ability to swallow. He believes that tubefeeding is to be classified as medical treatment and, as such, may be withheld on the grounds that it provides insufficient benefit and causes distress and suffering to patients; the ways in which it may do so are well explained in his paper.

Horan discusses withholding tubefeeding but does not consider the *withdrawing* of already initiated tubefeeding as a possibly distinct kind of choice. And yet it is not just obvious that the difference between withholding and withdrawing is in all circumstances morally insignificant. For a doctor may say (as Horan in effect does) that he is withholding tubefeeding because he is not obliged to employ *medical* means to strive to prolong a life when that life is irreversibly declining and the means to be employed are very likely to be burdensome to the patient. That being his reasoning, it is clear that a decision to withhold tubefeeding is not *aimed at* hastening the patient's death. It is a decision to refrain from doing what one believes one has no obligation to do, even though it is certain that death will be hastened by the decision.

But if we suppose tubefeeding to be established in a conscious, incompetent patient, withdrawal of it would require not just reasonable belief that at some point it is likely to prove seriously burdensome to the patient but clear evidence that it actually is so. If clear evidence of that kind did not exist what good reason would one have for ceasing to feed the patient? Once the tube is established there is nothing further to do *for the sake of feeding* than to keep on supplying the nutriment. And as long as the patient is not in the terminal phase of dying, what distinct reason could one have for stopping feeding which did not involve *intending* to starve the patient?

It is interesting that Joseph Boyle, in analysing and reflecting on the American debate about artificial nutrition and hydration, evidently does not think it relevant to distinguish between withholding and withdrawing, even though his discussion concentrates on patients in a persistent vegetative state (PVS). These are in a majority of instances accident victims, in whom tubefeeding would be established as a matter of course and in advance of establishing any accurate diagnosis of their condition. So in the normal course of events the question which arises in their care is whether to *withdraw* tubefeeding, not whether to withhold it. Since there is no very plausible case for saying that these patients are *suffering* from being tubefed, the question of whether one should continue to feed them may seem to raise exactly the same issue I identified in the previous paragraph in discussing tubefeeding of the *conscious*, incompetent patient who is not actually suffering from being tubefed. And in the case of such a patient there seemed to be no good reason for withdrawing tubefeeding.

But could it make no difference to the character of one's obligation that the PVS patient is said to be irreversibly unconscious? Clearly many participants in the discussion believe it makes a decisive difference. But Boyle shows that their reasons for saying so are not only ill-founded but imply the acceptability of hastening the deaths of more extensive groups of patients, such as the demented elderly. It is Boyle's examination of the *logic* of so much advocacy of withdrawing tubefeeding from PVS patients which makes his contribution relevant to a volume on the dependent elderly.

However, it is worth considering whether one evident difference between Horan and Boyle might suggest a less morally objectionable interpretation of the relevance of the *unconscious* state of PVS patients in determining whether or not one should withdraw tubefeeding from them. The difference I have in mind is that Horan thinks the fact that tubefeeding is *medical* treatment is morally significant, whereas Boyle believes that not much of moral significance can be made to hang on that claim. There is no discussion of the truth of Horan's view in the present volume, but it would be worth stating briefly the kind of case that might be made for it, and the kind of relevance it might be thought to have in determining the ethics of tubefeeding PVS patients.

Before doing so, however, one should note the significance for Boyle's view of the ethics of tubefeeding that he thinks nothing morally relevant is entailed by saying that tubefeeding is medical treatment. It follows that if one claims that tubefeeding of the PVS patient is *futile* one is not making some limited claim that tubefeeding is futile *qua* medical treatment; any such claim is to be interpreted as meaning that no benefit whatsoever could be secured by tubefeeding, and this seems to imply that the life of the PVS patient is without value.

Many do indeed believe that the lives of PVS patients lack value because they are incapable of significant experience and action. But, as Boyle points out, if this is true it would mean that the lives of other patients (such as those with advanced dementia or those who are severely retarded), who are incapable of significant experience and action, also lack value, Moreover, if it is reckoned that the lives of these patients lack value it becomes difficult to understand why one should not kill them, whether one seeks to accomplish that by withdrawing tubefeeding or in some other way. So it is clear why one influential line of argument to justify withdrawing tubefeeding from the PVS patients has large and radical implications for geriatric medicine.

Boyle is concerned to rebut the view that if a human being is incapable of significant experience and action he or she lacks value. One version of this view is that such human beings are as good as dead: they are incapable of a distinctively human life. They may be living human organisms but they are dead *qua* 'persons'. But, as Boyle remarks, the arguments for separating 'the idea of a human person from that of a living human organism are notoriously unpersuasive'. (For further on this point in the present volume see the contribution by John Finnis.)

Boyle thinks that the view that PVS patients cannot be benefited by having their lives prolonged is a second variant of the belief that human beings lack value who are incapable of significant experience and action. He therefore seeks to show both that persons can be benefited independently of their capacity to experience benefit, and that continued existence for the permanently unconscious is a benefit. The claim that it is not may rest on the belief that human life is merely instrumentally valuable (i.e. is valuable simply as a means to achieving some of the intrinsic goods which give point to human living) or, alternatively, on the belief that it is only contextually valuable (i.e. valuable in a context in which other intrinsic goods besides life itself are achievable). Boyle finds neither claim defensible, and concludes that the mere fact that a patient is permanently unconscious provides insufficient reason for withdrawing tubefeeding.

Withholding food and water undeniably causes death, but so does switching off a respirator when a patient is dependent on it. However, when respiratory support is judged medically otiose we do not think a doctor guilty of a person's death when he switches off the respirator on which that person has depended. He switches it off because it is otiose, not because he wishes to hasten the patient's death; the patient's death is not intended.

It is pretty clear, as Boyle indicates, that tubefeeding has been withdrawn in a number of cases precisely with the intention of hastening the deaths of PVS patients. Can it be withheld without one having that intention? Boyle thinks it certainly can, most clearly when the PVS patient, while still competent, had made a non-suicidal advance directive that he or she should not be fed if irreversibly comatose. A non-suicidal advance directive would be one aimed not precisely at bringing about one's own death but rather at some objective such as saving scarce medical resources so that they would be available for the care of others. To act in conformity with that kind of advance directive would be to cooperate with the patient's own authentic concern for human community and human solidarity.

But concern for human community and human solidarity is the main reason why, according to Boyle, tubefeeding should not be withdrawn from the majority of PVS patients. Tubefeeding is an expression of friendship and solidarity which cannot be denied with good reason to be beneficial to the PVS patient. To withdraw it in order to avoid costs, in the absence of advance directives to that effect, would be to abandon those patients, denying them that basic care which is only reasonably denied in the most exigent circumstances. Boyle does not believe those circumstances exist in the context of medical practice in the First World, so there is a moral obligation not to withdraw tubefeeding from the majority of PVS patients.

I remarked earlier that the present volume contains no developed defence of Michael Horan's view that tubefeeding is *medical* treatment and to his attaching moral significance to this classification of it. But it is not clear that someone who says that a doctor *qua* doctor has no obligation to seek to prolong a patient's life (even when the means necessary to prolong it are not burdensome to the patient) is thereby committed to saying that the life of that patient has either merely instrumental or merely contextual value. One's position might be that as a doctor one's obligation is to seek to restore health, i.e. some measure of bodily well-functioning. Accordingly the specific role and role-related duties of the doctor are to be understood in terms of the significance bodily well-functioning has in human life: certainly a good in itself (an intrinsic or basic good) but inextricably an instrumental good: a necessary means to the achieving of other intrinsic goods. Now, one may think that one does not know how a human being can be said to flourish to any degree if that person, *because of unconsciousness*, is incapable of realising, in however exiguous a measure, some intrinsic good besides organic well-functioning. And if one holds that the *raison d'etre* of the doctor is to make a specific kind of contribution to human flourishing (that of maintaining or restoring health or some approximation to it), then if the doctor finds himself unable to envisage what would count as the flourishing of a permanently unconscious patient, it is not clear that he can be under a role-related obligation to seek to prolong that patient's life.

Of course this position does depend on being able to show that there is a specific *raison d'etre* to medicine and specific duties attaching to the role of the doctor. (A doctor is not someone who by training has acquired a repertoire of technical skills which are arbitrarily called 'medical' and which he is obliged to employ to secure just any morally permissible benefits.) But if a doctor's duties are circumscribed by the character of his role, then a refusal to seek to prolong the life of a PVS patient need not be taken to imply that he regards the life of the PVS patient as lacking value. It may merely express the belief that he thinks it no part of a doctor's job to seek to prolong that life.

I have identified as one element in this position the statement that one does not know how a human being can be said to flourish if that person, because of permanent unconsciousness, is incapable of realising any good other than organic well-functioning. This should be taken strictly for what it is: a profession of *agnosticism*. It is certainly not a statement to the effect that a person incapable of significant experience and action lacks value. One may not know what could count as the flourishing of a PVS patient, and yet one could recognise, respect and reverence the dignity attaching to the humanity of that person. This would be shown by the fact that one regarded it as absolutely impermissible to seek to end that person's life.

The position sketched here remains undefended in the present volume, and the sketch offered is a long way from being the defence needed. Nonetheless, it does suggest how someone absolutely opposed to intentionally ending a patient's life might yet think that a doctor's circumscribed duty to seek to prolong life does not extend to the tubefeeding of certain patients for whom tubefeeding would not be directly burdensome.

Anyone wishing to argue this position would have to make a strong case for saying (a) that a doctor's duties are circumscribed in the way suggested, and (b) that one's obligations in regard to tubefeeding are of a strictly medical kind. In making such a case, one would have to take account of the eloquent and forceful case made by Boyle for saying that tubefeeding of PVS patients is in the majority of cases a basic requirement of friendship and solidarity with gravely deprived fellow human beings.

5

The Living Will: the ethical framework of a recent Report

LUKE GORMALLY

1 Introduction

The Living Will. Consent to Treatment at the End of Life[1] is the Report of a
Working Party established jointly by Age Concern England and The
Centre of Medical Law and Ethics of King's College, London. It was
published in 1988.

The Working Party of seven was chaired by Professor Ian Kennedy,
and, apart from the Director of Age Concern, was composed of three
doctors and three lawyers.

Their Report is undoubtedly the most important point of reference for
the discussion of advance directives in the British context. This discussion
has been given some degree of urgency by the advocacy of Living Wills
over a number of years by the Voluntary Euthanasia Society.

As one would expect from the composition of the Working Party, there
is much that is illuminating in the Report about medical practice and the
interpretation of English law. But the Report also aspires to offer an
ethical framework for advance directives.

After providing some information on parts of the Report which highlight the importance of its discussion of the ethics of advance directives
(section 2), I then go on to analyse what it has to say on this topic (section
3). Section 4 offers a critique of the ethical framework proposed by the
Report, and the final section (5) makes some summary observations on
the implications for public policy suggested by reflection on the Report's
proposed ethical underpinning of advance directives.

I have chosen to concentrate on the ethics of the Report not simply
because I possess no special competency to comment on its interpretation
of the law but, more importantly, because at the end of the day it is the
Report's conception of the ethical justification of advance directives and
of precisely what is held to be justified which are likely to prove most

influential. It is the proferred ethical justification which will be invoked by other advocates of living wills both as providing overall warrant and to defend the details of their proposals.

2 Some points in the report

2.1 The Report's view of the problem it is addressing

The Working Party's understanding of the essential background to the Report is stated in its opening sentences:

There are increasing numbers of incurably ill and incapacitated people, many of whom are elderly, who can be kept alive for prolonged periods by medical treatment and care, but who are incompetent to consent to or refuse such management. In recent years concern has been expressed that many of these people have received treatment which they would have refused if they had remained competent. This applies especially to new drugs and technologies and relates in particular to life sustaining treatment. (1)

The Report notes that two main reasons are advanced for concern about this situation:

The first is the desire to respect the liberty of individuals, and to protect them from the indignity, suffering and pain to which treatment may lead. The second relates to the social and economic costs, both to individual patients and families, and to the state, in looking after and treating large numbers of elderly and incapacitated people. The assumption in the second instance is that, given the opportunity to make their wishes known, a significant proportion of these people would opt for less or a different regime of treatment than is usually given with a consequent saving of resources. (1)

The Report very strongly identifies with the first of these concerns.[2] It proposes that an important and indispensable provision in meeting it should be the introduction of advance directives

whereby a person, whilst competent, specifically makes arrangements about his future health care decisions should he become incompetent. This may be achieved either by an instrument which has become known as a Living Will, or by a durable (or enduring) power of attorney (or a combination of both). (2)

The Report recognises that a correct understanding of what is required by the patient's 'best interests' 'would enable doctors to accept that there are instances where both ethically and legally it is already good practice to forgo further medical treatment.' But the Working Party is not convinced that it can be left to doctors to ensure that good practice of this kind prevails.

The Report is not in a position to draw on a broad range of empirical studies on how doctors in the UK treat the incompetent who are dying, debilitated or otherwise seriously impaired. One study is quoted for poor terminal care, with inadequate pain control. (12) But the Report's own account of Terminal Care (12–14) makes it clear that this situation is eminently remediable with proper training and the provision of resources.

The Report's relative lack of concern seriously to document the character of actual practice strengthens the impression that its authors share an *a priori* conviction either that it cannot be left to doctors to correct whatever is amiss in their treatment of the incompetent or that such correction would not satisfy some requirement of principle. The latter indeed seems to be the Working Party's view, for they share a dual conviction that (a) what is essentially at issue in deciding upon treatment for the incompetent is 'maximising respect for the liberty of individuals and autonomous decision making' (4) and (b) that this cannot be secured without a mechanism which ensures that paternalistic decision-making on behalf of the incompetent is kept to a minimum.[3]

2.2 Groups for whom advance directives are thought desirable

The Report envisages employment of advance directives in relation to three categories of patient:

those with terminal illness;

those with serious and permanent illness or disability who are not terminally ill but would die if not treated;

'Those with irreversible dementia who are not dying but who require long-term 24-hour care.' (8) Their treatment concerns 'matters of hygiene, feeding and medication to control the symptoms of their mental illness'. (9–10)

'For patients within each of these groups', the Working Party believes, 'there may come a time when both medically and ethically consideration should be given to withdrawing or withholding further treatment.' It should be noted that when the Report speaks of 'treatment' it includes artificially delivered nutrition and hydration. It claims that:

It is now acknowledged that artificial feeding and hydration, like any other treatment for the hopelessly ill patient [a phrase used to apply to all three categories of patient], should have a recognisable goal which is medically and ethically desirable. Any benefits need to be weighed carefully against the burdensome aspects for a particular patient. (20)

The Working Party believes that 'the most common condition in which some form of advance directive might be considered appropriate' is advanced dementia. 'By this means the individual would be able to retain some control over his life despite the onset of an incapacitating disease.' (17)

The Report holds that as a general rule an essential feature in assessing patients and determining treatment is evaluation of the patients' *quality of life*. The Working Party record a variety of views on the factors which should enter into a 'quality of life' judgement. They are inclined to say that which factors count most decisively must depend upon the outlook of each patient.

The Report clearly emphasises the need for much greater resources to be made available for the care of all three groups of patients. The impression that very clearly emerges from the Report is that the root difficulty over securing appropriate care for certain types of incompetent patient does not lie in medical attitudes. On the Report's own account it is doctors who have been largely responsible for the great improvements seen in recent decades in terminal care and geriatric care, and for the advances made recently, for example, in the more selective use of cardio-pulmonary resuscitation. Medical education has gradually become involved in the dissemination of these advances.

The root difficulty over securing appropriate care is not medical recalcitrance but the unavailability of the personnel and expertise which the Report indicates are required, particularly in the care of the elderly chronically ill and those suffering from dementia and brain damage. In circumstances in which patients are not well cared for not only do they deteriorate more rapidly than they might otherwise have done, but it is unsurprising if pressure builds to terminate the lives of those whose condition has become an embarrassment.

Despite the Report's view that resource considerations do not provide 'ethically respectable' reasons for advocating advance directives (47), it is important to be clear what is the most resistant source of the problem (of inappropriate care) which advance directives are supposed to be addressing. In our present economic circumstances, advance directives may well come to be seen as helping to solve a problem of badly funded care rather than a problem of unwarranted paternalism.

If there is truth in this observation then there is all the more reason to scrutinise carefully the ethical framework for advance directives which the Report proposes. Before doing so I shall briefly present that framework.

3 The Report's view of the ethical framework for advance directives

3.1 Preliminary remarks

Though Chapter 3 of the Report is entitled 'The Ethical and Legal Framework' there is no separate exposition of ethical principles. What is said about them emerges in the Report's analysis of legal principles. This makes for some obscurity about the Working Party's position, since it is not always clear whether it would be willing to offer an independent defence of the ethical principles identified, or whether those principles are presented precisely as the ethical assumptions which best make sense of English law. For present purposes the distinction does not perhaps greatly matter, since what is said in Chapter 3 about ethical principles is proposed as the normative framework for advance directives.

3.2 The exercise of the right of self-determination

Though it attracts little comment in Chapter 3, the Report is throughout shaped by the assumption that treatment decisions made in respect of incompetent patients should as far as possible take account of the principle of respect for patient autommy. This principle has its obvious application in the case of competent patients. But the Working Party believe that the exercise of self-determination by a competent patient in regard particularly to the withholding or withdrawing of treatment when he/she is incompetent ought normally to be respected as if it were a present exercise of self-determination by a competent patient. Self-determination on this account reaches beyond the loss of competency in the restraints it imposes on doctors and carers. Formal advance directives are desirable precisely in order to ensure that such self-determination is respected. In the absence of advance directives, the approach to be adopted by a proxy decision-maker 'should be that of "substituted judgement", rather than by reference to the patient's "best interests". In other words, the agent should attempt to be a sympathetic interpreter of the patient's wishes, rather than an objective judge of what would be in the patient's best interests.' (82) The rationale of 'substituted judgement' is that it is the closest approximation one can achieve to 'self-determination' by the patient in the absence of advance directives. Some authors even speak of exercising the right of self-determination on behalf of the patient!

3.3 The limits to self-determination through advance directives

The Report observes that English law about what is to be done in the case
of an incompetent patient whose wishes are unknown 'reflects and gives
effect to an ethical framework for medical practice within which all of the
problems we are considering fall to be analysed.' For 'English law recognises a legal justification for treating an incompetent patient where it is
necessary and *reasonable* to preserve or protect the patient's life or
health.' (37) These terms of reference suggest the question: When is it
neither necessary nor reasonable to preserve or protect life or health?

The following points are relevant to determining part of the Report's
answer to the question:

> it seems to be implied (at 38) that there is a quite general, morally
> significant distinction between acts and omissions.

> Consistent with this general thesis, the Working Party take the view
> that suicide cannot be accomplished by deliberate omission but that it
> requires one to carry out a positive act which directly causes one's own
> death. (29) Accordingly, they consider that a doctor cannot be said to
> assist suicide in withdrawing artificial nutrition and hydration.[4]

The fact that someone *now incompetent* determined while competent that
his life should be ended precisely by omission (either of medical treatment
or of food and fluids) in the kind of circumstances which now obtain is
never to be interpreted as a suicidal choice; for there is no such thing as
suicide by omission. So you *cannot* be given reason to seek to preserve life,
in the circumstances specified, by the thought that if you were to choose to
omit what is required for that purpose you would be aiding in suicide.

This crucially important feature of the Report's ethical framework does
not render other considerations irrelevant to determining the rightness or
wrongness of withholding treatment or food and fluids. The incompetent
patient you are now treating may not have made an advance directive or
may have made one which is insufficiently specific. In such circumstances
the Report purports to look for guidance to the traditional distinction
between 'ordinary' and 'extraordinary' means of preserving life. It quotes
the definition of these terms offered by a well-known American Catholic
moralist.[5] While it goes on, reasonably, to deprecate continued use of the
terms 'ordinary/extraordinary' because of the confusions associated with
them, it appears to wish to deploy the substance of the teaching those
terms were originally employed to articulate. What the Report offers as
an interpretation of that teaching is, however, radically at odds (as we

shall see) both with its presuppositions and its substance. This will be immediately clear, perhaps, from the following points the Report makes in expounding the teaching:

> the application of the teaching 'depends upon whether it is a good thing for the life to be prolonged'. (39, quoting Rachels[6])

> the substance of the distinction between 'ordinary' and 'extraordinary' is said to be 'in line with the third and objective test proposed by the *Conroy* court'. (40) According to the Report's own account of this test 'treatment could be withheld [in the absence of any evidence of the patient's wishes] only if it would clearly and markedly outweigh the benefits the patient derives from life'. (37)

> the distinction is held to be well elucidated by what the President's Commission said in interpreting it: 'extraordinary treatment is that which, in the patient's view, entails significantly greater burdens than benefits and is therefore undesirable and not obligatory, while ordinary treatment is that which, in the patient's view, produces greater benefits than burdens and is therefore reasonably desirable and undertaken.'[7]

The first two of these three glosses on the traditional teaching about ordinary and extraordinary means very clearly signal a shift from questions about the worthwhileness of *treatment* or the burdens of *treatment*, to questions about *the worthwhileness of a life* or the burdens of a life.

While, according to the Report, you may not perform an act intended to cause the death of an incompetent patient, you may follow a directive to omit treatment or artificial nutrition of such a patient when he had decided, while competent, that you should do so precisely because his condition makes his life no longer worthwhile in his eyes.

The straightforward implication of the Report's interpretation of the doctrine of ordinary and extraordinary means is that your proxy decision-maker may, under the guise of 'substituted judgement', decide that your life should be ended by omission of treatment because it is no longer worthwhile.

4 Critique of the Report's ethical framework

4.1 Incompetency and the right to self-determination

On what basis do we say that a person possesses a right to self-determination?[8] There are two elements to the basis.

First, human growth towards flourishing and fulfilment is essentially a matter of self-shaping through choices. So self-determination is an intrinsic and necessary feature of moral development and so of human flourishing.

Secondly, the exercise of the capacity for self-determination (and so of the right to self-determination) depends upon the development and continued possession of the following abilities:

that of understanding what kinds of choice make for human flourishing, and
that of choosing in a reasonable fashion.

If a person lacks these abilities, which constitute the capacity for self-determination, it does not make sense to *say* that he has a right to self-determination. As long as a person possesses the abilities, responsibility for what he makes of his life belongs *necessarily*, in the nature of moral agency, to him. But a person who loses these abilities, at least in regard to certain kinds of decision, *ipso facto* loses the capacity for self-determination in those matters. In those circumstances it is a deceptive fiction to speak of that person *possessing* the right to self-determination.

When a person loses the capacity for self-determination, either wholly or relative to certain kinds of decision, then some other person or persons must take responsibility for the now incompetent person. In that situation it is at best misconceived, and therefore confusing, to speak of those with responsibility as exercising the incompetent person's right to self-determination. He no longer has such a right. The responsibility for what becomes of him rests squarely on others.

In reflecting on that responsibility of proxy decision-makers we need to bear in mind that the point and purpose of the exercise of self-determination (which has now been replaced by the proxy's choosing) was the flourishing of the subject. Similarly, the point and purpose of the proxy's choosing must be the flourishing of the now incompetent subject i.e. that person's good. And to serve that person's good the proxy's choices must at the very least conform to the requirements of justice.

4.2 *The supposed binding force of advance directives*

Buchanan and Brock, in their large-scale study of our topic,[9] have sought to show that if there is reason to respect the wishes of the dead, there must be stronger reason to respect the interests of the incompetent as determined by themselves when competent.

There is indeed reason to respect the wishes of a person now dead *in regard to his property* just because it was his to dispose of. But it is different with a man's body even when that is no longer the body of a living person but a corpse. If a man stipulated in his will that after death his body should be roasted at a feast and his friends should eat it (to signify communion with him) we should reject his wishes (a) because it is not open to him to dispose of his body in the way that it would be open to him to dispose of his herd of fatted calves, and (b) because what he stipulated is contrary to the respect owing to the human body, a respect we connect with the dignity of the human (bodily) person.

A fortiori (one may certainly say), there are limits on the determination by a competent person of what should happen to him should be become incompetent. Those limits are dictated by similar considerations: a man's bodily life is not a disposable piece of property; an incompetent person is a living human being, who possesses a dignity which excludes our treating that person in certain ways.

It seems clear, then, that the analogy with *post mortem* implementation of a man's will suggests, if anything, that there must be normative constraints on implementation of advance directives.

No one thinks that an advance directive in regard to medical treatment is like a marriage vow – that it binds the person who makes it to some unalterable commitment which others should respect as such. In all jurisdictions that recognise advance directives they are revocable *at any time* by a competent person making them.

This fact implicitly recognises that a person may have reason to change his mind about future treatment. If there is a good reason for a person to change his mind then someone who was truly a friend would certainly want to persuade that person to make the change. An incompetent person, however, in the nature of his condition is not open to being rationally persuaded to a change of mind. Why, in these circumstances, should one treat as immutable a prior directive which any true friend of the person who made it would regard as seriously misguided? To do so does not show respect for the now incompetent patient; on the contrary he is disadvantaged by being treated as captive to his prior folly.

When a person while competent has chosen to be treated in ways which are contrary to his dignity as a human being, we should not respect those decisions when he becomes incompetent; because it is consistent neither with justice nor friendship to treat a person in ways which are inconsistent with recognition of his dignity as a human being.

The question of what is and what is not consistent with respect for human dignity is addressed in 4.4 below. In concluding this section it is worth noting that what is characteristically missing in much modern discussion of autonomy and self-determination is any strong sense that the most fundamental expression of respect for the dignity of human beings is *not* respect for autonomy but rather respect for the *good* of human beings. When persons have *exercisable capacities* for self-determination then respect for self-determination (or autonomy) is integral to respect for their good as persons: for it is *through choice* that they have the possibility of shaping their characters for good (or ill). But when persons do not yet, or no longer, possess presently exercisable capacities for self-determination, self-determination cannot be an essential ingredient, so to speak, in what we respect in respecting their good. Any exercise of self-determination which seeks to determine what should (or should not) happen to one when one is incompetent should be respected *only to the extent that doing so is consistent with respecting the good of the now incompetent patient.*

4.3 Acts, omissions and killing[10]

As we saw (3.3 above) the Report seems to assume that there is a quite general, morally significant distinction between acts and omissions. This is to adopt a position opposite to that of utilitarians who characteristically think that no morally significant distinction can be drawn between acts and omissions. What counts for a utilitarian in the moral evaluation of choice are the *foreseeable* consequences of one's choice, whether the choice be to do something or to omit to do something.

By contrast with both views the tradition of common morality draws a morally significant distinction between intended and foreseen consequences.[11] One commits oneself to the intended results of one's chosen actions or omissions in a way in which one is not in general committed to the foreseen consequences of one's actions or omissions. It is in the nature of that commitment to be character-shaping and therefore of crucial moral significance.

One can aim at (i.e. intend) a person's death either by chosen actions or by chosen omissions.

It is surprising that these truths are not recognised by the Working Party, for two reasons at least.

First, the Working Party hold that it is morally and legally acceptable to act with sufficient reason in a way which causes bad side-effects; e.g. it is acceptable to seek to control pain with drugs which have the unintended effect of hastening the death of the patient, because the relief of pain is a 'lawful purpose' (38). But the doctrine of double effect accepted by the Working Party does not make much sense without recognition of the moral significance of the distinction between intended and foreseen consequences of choice.

Secondly, English law (a prime source of moral insight for the Working Party) recognises that there can be murder by a course of omissions intended to cause death.[12]

The Report seeks to assure doctors that they cannot be guilty of assisting suicide in withdrawing life-prolonging treatment or artificially delivered food and fluids because suicide cannot be committed by deliberate omission.

It ought to be clear that, morally speaking, suicide, just like murder, can be accomplished by omission.

But to talk of 'assisting suicide' in the context of treating the incompetent is in any case confused. If the incompetent do not possess the capacity for reasoned choice (and so lack in any defensible sense a right to self-determination) then they are not in a position to decide to kill themselves. A doctor who decides to kill an incompetent patient – whether by act or omission – in the confused belief that he is assisting in suicide is doing no such thing. What he is engaged in is much more like murder.

Nothing that I have said by way of clarifying the notions of 'act' and 'omission' should be taken to imply that doctors have an unqualified duty to prolong life. The Report holds such a conception of duty to be characteristic of 'the sanctity of life' ethic, but it has to be said that the Report is seriously irresponsible in its interpretation of it. We can now turn to some brief clarification of a sanctity of life ethic in explaining the import of the traditional distinction between ordinary and extraordinary means of prolonging life.

4.4 Presuppositions of traditional teaching about ordinary and extraordinary means

At the end of 3.3 above I indicated that, though the Report purports to draw on the substance of the traditional teaching articulated in the distinction between ordinary and extraordinary means, it rather radically alters the import of that teaching. It is reinterpreted as encapsulating an answer to questions about the obligation to treat based not on the worthwhileness or burdens of *treatment* but rather on the worthwhileness or burdens of a life.

This travesty is possible because of ignorance of the two basic assumptions of a sanctity of life ethic in its bearings on the practice of medicine.

The first assumption is that all human beings possess a dignity, *just in virtue of being human*, of a kind which is incompatible with our killing a human being on the basis of a judgement that he lacks a worthwhile life. This assumption is quite fundamental to the order of justice in society. (For a brief explanation of this assumption see my chapter: 'The Aged: non-persons, human dignity and justice', in this volume.)

The second assumption crucial to a sanctity of life ethic in medicine is that prolongation of life is not *per se* an objective of medical practice. The primary purpose of medical care is the restoration and preservation of health; it exists to serve the good of health. By health I understand that condition of the body in virtue of which it functions well as an organic whole, so that the individual enjoys physical vitality in itself and thereby is also well-placed to achieve some of the other goods of human fulfilment.[13]

Medical efforts to prolong a life which would otherwise come to an end are in general justifiable only in so far as a patient has some continuing capacity for integrated organic functioning *sufficient* to allow him to continue to share in some of the other goods of human life (e.g. contemplation of truth or beauty, friendship, including the experience of the affection and care of others, the exercise of choice, prayer, play).

It is a mistake, leading to much confusion, to believe that prolongation of life is an independent aim of medical care.[14]

The core of a sanctity of life ethic is an exceptionless negative prohibition on intentionally killing innocent human beings. It involves no exceptionless positive obligation (if *per impossibile* such could exist[15]) to prolong life.

It is perfectly possible, therefore, within a sanctity of life ethic, to ask when it is reasonable not to seek *medically* to prolong life. The considerations which are centrally relevant to answering that question concern

(i) the likelihood of treatment being successful in prolonging a life sufficiently approximating to health to allow participation in some other basic aspect of human flourishing, and

(ii) the extent of the burdensome consequences for living which result from treatment.

Treatment which offers little prospect of success or which creates undue burdens for the patient is not treatment which he is obliged to undergo or which a doctor is obliged to offer (viz. it is 'extraordinary'); treatment which is likely to be successful and does not create undue burdens is treatment which a doctor ought to offer and which a competent patient ought to accept (viz. it is 'ordinary').[16]

Since what will count as unduly burdensome will depend to some extent on the condition and characteristic sensibility and sensitivity of each individual patient, then it is indeed important in treating the incompetent to have reliable information about which predictable consequences of treatment they are likely to find very burdensome. It may therefore be useful to have written declarations from people while competent on the outcomes of treatment which they anticipate would bear heavily upon them. But even such declarations cannot be thought to have any kind of binding authority, since impairment and incompetence may alter the outlook and expectations of a patient. So those responsible for the care of the incompetent must make an independent judgement about what is in the best interests of that patient.

What cannot be even *considered* to be in the best interests of a patient is that one should seek to end his life because one judges that life no longer worthwhile. The ethical framework of the Report on *The Living Will* is seriously defective just because it makes the choice to behave in that way seem a reasonable option in certain circumstances.

5 Concluding reflections: the ethics of the Report and public policy

5.1 Four points

There is much that could be said under the general heading of the final part of this chapter but I shall have to confine myself to a number of summary observations.

First, as a matter of public policy there is an urgent need that the practice of medicine should not undermine the moral integrity of doctors. But moral integrity would be undermined by any requirement that doctors should seek to end lives by withholding treatment on the authority of an advance directive indicating that the patient's present condition renders his life no longer worthwhile.

Secondly, if such a practice were authorised it would amount to the practice of non-voluntary euthanasia. If non-voluntary euthanasia by omission is permissible then there will be no grounds consistent with this position for prohibiting non-voluntary euthanasia carried out by some positive act. Indeed there will be many circumstances in which active euthanasia is likely to seem more merciful and humane than euthanasia

by, for example, starvation. Proponents of the legalization of active
euthanasia have from time to time suggested they might succeed in their
efforts precisely on the basis of the perception that active euthanasia is
more humane than euthanasia by omission.[17] The latter they hope to see
accepted through acceptance of living wills. The ethical framework of the
Report on *The Living Will* readily accommodates euthanasia by omission.

Thirdly, it seems very likely in present circumstances (with the heavy
emphasis on cost containment in the provision of health care) that, if
living wills come to have the authority their advocates desire, pressure will
be exerted on individuals to complete them precisely with a view to cost
containment and in a form conducive to cost containment. The Report
itself repudiates this as a reason for expecting people to make advance
directives. (47) But like many advocates of social change, the members of
the Working Party fail to recognise that once a change is initiated its
potential 'benefits' will not remain to be controlled by the individuals who
initiated the change under a limited and specific conception of its benefits.

Fourthly, as I remarked in section 2.2, the root difficulty over securing
good quality care of the categories of patient which concern the Working
Party stems from failures to make personnel and expertise available.
These failures, of course, reflect the low esteem in which certain groups of
patients are held, and are not motivated by 'purely economic' considerations. To propose a framework for advance directives in which it is
acceptable to end the lives of patients because they are believed no longer
to have worthwhile lives can only serve to reinforce the low esteem in
which such patients are held. This will make it all the more likely that
advance directives are exploited to evade the need to improve clinical
care. We should be placing emphasis on improving care, which certainly
includes improving the sensitivity and ethical integrity of doctors and
nurses. We need doctors with a proper conception of the limited good
they are qualified to secure for patients and a proper conception of when
they should cease to strive to prolong life. Patients could not be well-
served by any arrangement which compromises that respect for human
dignity which is the foundation of justice and an indispensable presuppo-
sition of clinical practice.

5.2 *'Autonomy' and the prospective fate of the incompetent*

I find it difficult to avoid the impression that much of the talk in
bioethics about autonomy (highly incongruous talk in relation to the
incompetent) generates a smokescreen to obscure what is really going

forward in the social transformation of medicine in our society. By way of conclusion let me explain why.

The predominant theoretical context of the discussion about treatment decisions (at least in Anglo-Saxon countries) is provided by liberalism and liberalism's aversion to paternalism. However, classical liberalism for the most part thought paternalistic treatment of the incompetent appropriate.

Modern versions of liberalism, however, affect to find something objectionable about paternalistic treatment of the incompetent. Why this change? In part it stems from a deeper contemporary scepticism about what to count as making for the well-being of the incompetent.[18] But it also appears to stem from a perverse perception of many of the incompetent as no longer possessing worthwhile lives[19], so that it becomes plausible to say either that, if they had their wits about them, they would realise they would be better off dead ('substituted judgement' approach), or that, since they so little approximate to being persons, they can no longer be considered to possess the normal person's interest in continued existence ('best interests' approach).

So contemporary liberalism, despite protestations to the contrary, devises an ideology in which it no longer seems absolutely forbidden to rid ourselves of those patients – particularly the debilitated and demented elderly – who increasingly are perceived as an unacceptable burden on the health care budget. Contemporary bioethics is a rich source of such rationalizations of convenience. I fear that *The Living Will* relies on an 'ethical framework' which is all too likely to prove fertile in rationalizations for disposing of the incompetent rather than upholding their dignity.

Notes

1 *The Living Will. Consent to Treatment at the End of Life.* A Working Party Report. London: Edward Arnold 1988. Arabic numbers in brackets in the present chapter refer to pages of the Report.

2 The validity of the second concern is recognised by the Working Party. In discussing judgements about what counts as good medical practice, the only *objective* element in such judgements explicitly identified by the Report is seen as a function of the limits that resources impose on satisfying the demands of individual patients (79–80). (It should be observed that such limits are contingent, and do not suggest any substantive norms of good medical practice.) Despite its view that consideration of resources serves to give an element of objectivity to judgements about treatment, the Report (at 47) considers the desire to save resources does not provide 'an ethically respectable reason for advocating' advance directives. This viewpoint is completely consistent with the Working Party's view that there should be minimal constraints on self-determination in the formulation of advance directives.

3 One important question which reflection on the Report suggests is whether

there is a sound defence for speaking, in regard to treatment of incompetent patients, of 'maximising respect for the *liberty* of individuals and *autonomous* decision-making'. I shall return to this in discussing the Report's ethical framework at 4.1.

4 The Report goes on to say that: 'While United States law in this area is heavily dependent upon constitutional rights, particularly the right of privacy, we believe English law would reflect the approach of the *Bouvia* case basing itself upon the need for consent to treat which is itself based upon the ethical obligation to respect the individual's autonomy . . .' (29–30) To a non-lawyer the view that English law would reflect *Bouvia* seems both amazing and alarming. Would it go so far as to reflect Judge Lynn Compton's concurring opinion in *Bouvia* in which straightforward assistance in suicide is presented as not merely legitimate for doctors but a duty of theirs? See especially the following:

'Elizabeth [Bouvia] apparently has made a conscious and informed choice that she prefers death to continued existence in her helpless and, to her, intolerable condition. I believe that she has an absolute right to effectuate that decision. This State and the medical profession, instead of frustrating her desire, should be attempting to relieve her suffering by permitting and in fact assisting her to die with ease and dignity. The fact that she is forced to suffer the ordeal of self-starvation to achieve her objective is in itself inhumane.'

'The right to die is an integral part of our right to control our own destinies so long as the rights of others are not affected. That right should, in my opinion, include the ability to enlist the assistance from others, including the medical profession, in making death as quick and painless as possible.' (Quoted in Robert L. Barry, *Medical Ethics. Essays on Abortion and Euthanasia* New York: Peter Lang 1989, 101–2.)

5 'Ordinary means are all medicines, treatments and operations which offer a reasonable hope of benefit for the patient and which can be obtained and used without excessive expense, pain or other inconvenience. On the other hand extraordinary means are all medicines, treatments and operations which cannot be obtained or used without excessive expense, pain or other inconvenience, or which, if used, would not offer a reasonable hope of benefit.' (38–9, quoting the late Gerald Kelly SJ, *Medico-Moral Problems* St Louis: The Catholic Hospital Association 1958, 129. Kelly's definitions purport to summarise long-standing usage of the terms in Catholic moral theology.)

6 The choice of James Rachels as an interpreter of the traditional distinction is perhaps symptomatic, for he is plainly hostile to its rationale and import as traditionally understood.

7 President's Commission for the Study of Ethical Problems in Medicine and Biomedical and Behavioral Research, *Deciding to Forego Life-Sustaining Treatment. A Report on the Ethical, Medical and Legal Issues in Treatment Decisions* Washington, D.C., 1983, 88. Two points should be made about this quotation from the Commission's Study. First, 'ordinary' treatment, as traditionally understood, is treatment which is *obligatory*, not just treatment which is 'reasonably desirable and undertaken'. Secondly, the ordinary/extraordinary distinction cannot be explained by reference to a wholly *subjective* viewpoint. It is true that a judgement on how burdensome the consequences of treatment are must depend upon the condition and sensibility of the patient. But it is not open to the patient simply to *decide* what is to count as a benefit of treatment.

8 For further observations on self-determination or autonomy see my Introduction to this volume.

9 Allen E. Buchanan and Dan W. Brock, *Deciding for Others: The Ethics of Surrogate Decision Making* Cambridge: Cambridge University Press 1989.

10 See further [Luke Gormally] *Is there a morally significant difference between killing and letting die?* London: The Linacre Centre 1978.

11 The facts of moral psychology which make this distinction intelligible are briefly stated in Luke Gormally, Euthanasia: some points in a philosophical polemic, in *Death without Dignity. Euthanasia in Perspective* ed. N. Cameron, Edinburgh: Rutherford House Books 1990, 47–65; see especially 58–60. The same paper appears in *The Linacre Quarterly* (USA) 57/2 (May 1990), 14–25.

12 The principal authority for this is *R v. Gibbons and Proctor* (1981) 13 Cr.App.R.134, especially at 137–8. See the lengthy note 2 of the article cited in the previous note, 63–64.

13 It will be evident that I fairly closely align myself with the position of Leon Kass in his essay 'Regarding the end of medicine and the pursuit of health', *The Public Interest* 40 (Summer 1975), 11–42; reprinted in *Concepts of Health and Disease. Interdisciplinary Perspectives* ed. A. L. Caplan, H. T. Engelhardt, and J. J. McCartney, 3–30. Reading, Mass: Wiley, 1981.

14 The last three paragraphs follow closely parts of section 3 of Luke Gormally, A response [to Roy Fox, Palliative care and aggressive therapy], in *Medical Ethics and Elderly People* ed. R. John Elford, 177–98. Edinburgh: Churchill Livingstone, 1987.

15 There cannot be exceptionless obligations *to act* in such and such a way.

16 A fairly full exposition of traditional teaching may be found in [Luke Gormally] *Ordinary and extraordinary means of prolonging life*. London: The Linacre Centre, 1979. A more consise explanation is offered in section 6 of the paper referred to in note 14, (at 194–6).

17 As exemplified by the following statement made by Helga Kuhse of the Centre for Human Bioethics, Monash University, Melbourne: 'If we can get people to accept the removal of all treatment and care – especially the removal of food and fluids – they will see what a painful way this is to die, and then, in the patient's best interest, they will accept the lethal injection.' The statement was made in a panel discussion on 21 September 1984 at the Fifth Biennial Conference of the World Federation of Right to Die Societies, Nice, France, 20–23 September 1984; it is reported in Rita Marker, The ethical values that civil law must respect in the field of euthanasia, *The Linacre Quarterly* (USA) 56/3 (August 1989), 22–35.

18 On the roots of modern moral scepticism see Alasdair MacIntyre, *After Virtue*. London: Duckworth and Notre Dame: Notre Dame University Press, 1981; 2nd edn. 1984.

19 On which see further my chapter, The aged: non-persons, human dignity and justice, in the present volume.

6

Some reflections on euthanasia in The Netherlands

JOHN KEOWN

Introduction

Drawing on empirical research which I have been carrying out in The Netherlands since 1989,[1] this paper examines critically the Dutch euthanasia experience.

Part I deals with the offence of taking a person's life at his request contained in article 293 of the Penal Code and the extent to which the courts have allowed doctors a defence to this charge. Part II considers the guidelines for voluntary euthanasia which have been set out by the Royal Dutch Medical Association (KNMG). Part III examines the extent to which the Dutch experiment confirms or confutes a major ethical argument against the legalisation of voluntary euthanasia, namely, the 'slippery slope' argument.

Part I: The offence of killing a person at his request and the defence of necessity

1 The offence of killing a person at his request

Killing a person at his 'express and serious request' is punished by article 293 of the Penal Code.[2] It is one of the 'Serious offences against human life'[3] in Title XIX of the Code. Article 287 provides that a person who intentionally takes another's life without premeditation commits 'homicide'[4], but a person who intentionally and with premeditation takes the life of another is guilty of murder: article 289.[5]

Article 294 punishes assisting suicide.[6] Suicide itself is not criminal; nor is aiding attempted suicide, evidently because the legislature feared that the imposition of criminal liability might encourage a further attempt.[7]

In short, voluntary euthanasia, or the intentional acceleration of a patient's death at his request as part of his medical care, is prohibited by article 293. The intentional killing of an incompetent person (non-voluntary euthanasia) or of a person against his wishes (involuntary euthanasia) would constitute either murder (contrary to article 289) or 'homicide' (contrary to article 287).

2 *The defence of necessity*

(i) *The Supreme Court decision of 1984*

Notwithstanding the apparently clear terms of article 293, the criminal courts have come to interpret the Code as providing a defence to a charge of voluntary euthanasia under that article and equally to a charge of assisting suicide under article 294. The line of relevant cases stretches from the decision of a District Court in 1973 to decisions of the Supreme Court in 1984 and 1986.[8]

The Supreme Court decision of 27 November 1984, the *Alkmaar* case, involved the killing of an elderly woman, a 'Mrs B', at her request by her GP. The doctor was acquitted by the Alkmaar District Court but, on an appeal by the prosecution, was convicted by the Court of Appeal at Amsterdam. He then appealed successfully to the Supreme Court[9] which held that the Court of Appeal had wrongly rejected the doctor's defence that he had acted out of necessity. The Supreme Court held that the Court of Appeal had not given sufficient reasons for its decision and that, in particular, it should have investigated whether 'according to responsible medical opinion' measured by the 'prevailing standards of medical ethics' a situation of necessity existed.[10]

The defence of necessity is contained in article 40 of the Penal Code, which provides that a person who commits an offence as a result of 'irresistible compulsion or necessity [*overmacht*] is not criminally liable'.[11] The defence takes two forms: first, 'psychological compulsion' and secondly 'emergency' (*noodtoestand*) or choosing to break the law in order to promote a higher good.[12] Commenting on the latter form of the defence as applied by the Supreme Court to euthanasia, Professor Mulder, an expert on criminal law, explains that it refers to the situation where a doctor, faced with the dire distress of his patient, is faced with a 'conflict of interests' which results in the doctor breaking the law to promote a higher good.[13]

The Supreme Court observed in the *Alkmaar* case that whether a situation of necessity existed would depend on the circumstances of the case and that the Appeal Court could have taken into account, for example, the following matters:

whether and to what extent according to professional medical judgement an increasing disfigurement of the patient's personality and/or further deterioration of her already unbearable suffering were to be expected;

whether it could be expected that soon she would no longer be able to die with dignity under circumstances worthy of a human being;

whether there were still opportunities to alleviate her suffering.[14]

The case was referred to the Hague Court of Appeal with a direction that it investigate whether, on the facts, the performance of euthanasia by the doctor 'would, *from an objective medical perspective*, be regarded as an action justified in a situation of necessity'.[15] On 11 September 1986, the Court of Appeal acquitted the accused on the basis that the defence of necessity applied.[16] Having noted that the accused maintained that he had done nothing contrary to medical ethics, the Court added that he had, on the basis of his expertise as a physician and his experience as Mrs. B's doctor, and after careful consideration of conflicting duties in the light of medical ethics, made a choice which had to be regarded as justified according to 'reasonable' medical opinion.[17] Advocate-General Feber has noted the substitution of 'reasonable' for 'objective' medical opinion[18] and that the Court raised for discussion the question of the degree to which euthanasia could be justified by a normal psychological reaction to physical deterioration.[19]

(ii) The Supreme Court decision of 1986

On 21 October 1986, one month after the decision of the Hague Court of Appeal, the Supreme Court delivered a second judgment on euthanasia.[20] This case[21] concerned the prosecution of a doctor who, after repeated requests, euthanatised a 73 year-old friend suffering from advanced multiple sclerosis. The doctor was convicted by the Groningen District Court and her conviction was upheld by the Court of Appeal at Leeuwarden. The Supreme Court, however, allowed her appeal, holding that the Court of Appeal had wrongly failed to consider two defences raised at trial. The first was that the accused acted because of her patient's 'dire distress'; the second that she acted out of 'psychological necessity' because she 'was confronted with the suffering of her patient and found *herself* under duress and could not arrive at any other decision than to grant the assistance requested'.[22] The Supreme Court remitted the case to the Court of Appeal at Arnhem for further investigation[23]; the doctor was convicted.[24]

(iii) The criteria for lawful euthanasia: a summary

The criteria laid down by the courts to determine whether the defence of necessity applies in a given case of euthanasia have been summarised by Mrs Borst-Eilers, Vice-President of the Health Council (a body which provides scientific advice to the Government on health issues), as follows:

1 The request for euthanasia must come only from the patient and must be entirely free and voluntary.
2 The patient's request must be well considered, durable and persistent.
3 The patient must be experiencing intolerable (not necessarily physical) suffering, with no prospect of improvement.
4 Euthanasia must be a last resort. Other alternatives to alleviate the patient's situation must have been considered and found wanting.
5 Euthanasia must be performed by a physician.
6 The physician must consult with an independent physician colleague who has experience in this field.[25]

Whether consultation must be with an 'independent' physician is, however, doubtful; in the *Alkmaar* case the defendant GP had merely consulted his assistant. Further, it has been pointed out by Eugene Sutorius, counsel to the Dutch Voluntary Euthanasia Society (DVES), that the Supreme Court has stated that consultation is not always essential. He has explained that, although the Court did not elaborate on this point, in his view, as the purpose of consultation is to obtain a second opinion about the medical aspects of the case, consultation is not necessary when there is no doubt about these aspects and when witnesses are available to verify that the non-medical criteria have been satisfied.[26]

(iv) Liability for falsifying the death certificate

Necessity is not, however, a defence to a charge of falsely certifying the cause of death. In a case decided by the Court of the Hague (Penal Chamber) in 1987, the defendant doctor admitted that, having performed euthanasia, he had certified that death was due to natural causes[27]. The Court of Appeal upheld the trial court's decision that death by euthanasia was not death by natural causes and that the doctor could not rely on necessity as a defence to falsifying the death certificate. The Appeal Court declared that it was a matter of great public concern that non-natural

deaths should be investigated by officials such as the coroner and prosecutor and that this was especially so in cases of euthanasia in view of the
proven danger of abuse.[28]

Part II: Medical Guidelines

The judgment of the Hague Court of Appeal in the *Alkmaar* case gave
striking weight to the views of a 'considerable number of medical doctors'
against whom, it said, a judge could not 'make a choice in this matter'.[29]
In fact, the medical profession, or at least its main representative body,
the Royal Dutch Medical Association (KNMG), to which some 60% of
the 30 000 Dutch doctors belong, has played a significant role in the
relaxation of the law and practice of euthanasia.

1 The KNMG Criteria

In 1973 the KNMG issued a provisional statement which said that
euthanasia should remain a crime but that if a doctor shortened the life of
a patient who was incurably ill and in the process of dying, a court would
have to judge whether there was not a conflict of duties which justified the
doctor's action.[30] In August 1984, three months before the decision of the
Supreme Court in the *Alkmaar* case, the central committee of the KNMG
produced a Report setting out the criteria which the KNMG felt should
be satisfied in cases of euthanasia.[31] As Borst-Eilers has pointed out, there
is a close correspondence between these criteria and those laid down by
the courts.[32] Subsequently, the KMNG formulated[33] certain 'Guidelines
for Euthanasia'.[34]

The Report lists five criteria: 'voluntariness'; 'a well-considered
request'; 'a durable death-wish'; 'unacceptable suffering', and 'consultation between colleagues'[35]. These are reproduced in the Guidelines.[36]

(i) Voluntariness

The Report stresses that the request must be made of the patient's free will
and must not be the result of pressure by others.[37] Conceding that it will
not always be possible to be completely sure that the request is not
influenced by others, the Report says that the doctor should talk privately
with the patient and that, after a 'number of conversations', he must be
able to get a 'fairly reliable impression' of the voluntariness of the
request.[38] The Guidelines, by contrast, state that there need only be 'a'
conversation with the patient to verify voluntariness.[39]

(ii) A well-considered request

To ensure that the request is well-considered the Report urges that the doctor should give the patient a 'clear picture of his medical situation and the appropriate prognosis' and, because a request for euthanasia is 'not uncommonly found to be an expression of fear – such as fear of pain, deterioration, loneliness' the doctor should also examine the extent to which these fears influence the request, and should dispel them as far as possible.[40]

Similarly, the Guidelines state that a doctor must guard against granting a request which arises essentially from 'other problems than the will to terminate life' such as the feeling of being superfluous or a nuisance to the family. A request made on such grounds should first of all be an occasion for a consultation with the patient about alternative solutions; in no case should euthanasia be granted because of problems which could be resolved in another way.[41]

(iii) A durable death wish

The Report declares that requests arising out of 'impulse or a temporary depression' should not be granted but adds that it is not possible to indicate what time span should have elapsed before a request becomes 'durable'.[42] The physician is advised to 'steer mostly by his own compass' but that 'durable', in the opinion of the committee, does not simply mean more than once.[43]

(iv) Unacceptable suffering

The Guidelines state that the patient must experience his suffering as 'persistent, unbearable, and hopeless' and they add that the relevant case-law indicates that an important consideration is whether the patient will be able to die 'in a dignified manner'.[44]

The Report, however, states that the committee, while aware that the courts indicated that the suffering must be persistent, unbearable and hopeless, declined to support this definition of the criterion because it felt that these concepts overlapped and were unverifiable.[45] It continues that although the degree of suffering is an important criterion, there are only limited possibilities for verification since the unbearable and hopeless character of a person's situation is so dependent on individual standards and values that an objective assessment is difficult.[46]

Suffering, says the Report, can have any of three causes: first, pain; secondly, a physical condition or physical disintegration without pain; and thirdly, suffering without any physical complaint which could be caused either by 'social factors and the like' in a healthy person or by a 'medical-psychiatric syndrome'.[47] Pain, the Report continues, can be controlled to such an extent that, in general, it is not a primary cause of unbearable suffering. And as to suffering caused by social factors, a doctor usually cannot assess the unbearability of the patient's situation or the prospects of its alleviation.[48]

The Report adds that, although the KNMG's 1973 statement had raised the question whether euthanasia was justifiable if the patient were incurably ill and in the process of dying,[49] the committee felt that, quite apart from the fact that the 'dying phase' could not be clearly defined, it was not reasonable to deny a patient who was suffering unbearably the 'right to euthanasia' solely because he was not dying. Consequently, it could no longer support the 'dying phase' as a criterion.[50]

(v) Consultation and reporting

The committee considered consultation with a colleague with experience in this field to be 'indispensable' to promote well-balanced decision-making[51] and the Report recommends that the doctor consult first a colleague with whom he is professionally involved and later an independent doctor.[52]

Finally, having noted that it was 'not unusual' for cases of euthanasia to be reported as a natural death in order to protect the relatives and/or the doctor from police investigation, the Report urges that this 'improper' practice be discontinued and stresses the committee's advocacy of due openness in the reporting of death.[53]

2 Current Medical and Legal Procedures

Procedures followed by doctors who have performed euthanasia vary throughout the country. At one of the leading centres for euthanasia, the Reinier de Graaf Hospital in Delft, the procedure is that the doctor does not certify a natural death but informs the police.[54] The municipal medical examiner comes to inspect the body and a policeman to interview the doctor. Both officials then file reports with the prosecutor who, if satisfied that the legal criteria have been met, gives permission for the corpse to be handed over to the relatives.[55] As Borst-Eilers comments: 'This whole procedure after death need only take a few hours. Only if the public prosecutor suspects that all the criteria have not been met with, he orders further interviews with nurses, members of the family etc.'[56] If the prosecutor's suspicions are not allayed, he may then ask an examining magistrate to investigate. In November 1990, however, the Minister of Justice and KNMG agreed that the doctor need only report to the medical examiner, and the Minister of Justice directed prosecutors that on receiving the examiner's report they should ask the police to investigate euthanasia cases only when there are grounds for suspecting that the appropriate criteria have not been met.[57]

The final decision whether to prosecute is taken at a meeting of the country's five Chief Prosecutors (*Procureurs-Generaal*) according to the criteria laid down by the courts. The Chief Prosecutors, each of whom is attached to one of the five regional Courts of Appeal, meet every three weeks, together with a representative from the Ministry of Justice, to discuss prosecution policy in relation to crimes in general and to decide, according to the criteria laid down by the courts,[58] whether to prosecute in each notified case of euthanasia. In practice, they simply approve the decision of the local prosecutor.[59]

Part III: Sliding Down a Slippery Slope?

Having set out in Part I the legal and in Part II the medical criteria for voluntary euthanasia, I can now examine the extent to which the experience of euthanasia in The Netherlands confirms or confutes the 'slippery slope' argument, an argument which has been deployed in major reports opposing the legalisation of voluntary euthanasia, such as those of the Working Party of the Church of England's Board for Social Responsibility (1975),[60] the Canadian Law Reform Commission (1983),[61] and the Working Party of the British Medical Association (1988).[62] On this argument, even if euthanasia in certain circumstances (in particular that of a free and well-considered request by the patient) is not intrinsically wrong, its legalisation will result in a slide down a 'slippery slope' to non-voluntary and possibly even involuntary euthanasia. It will do so, the argument runs, either because any safeguards which might prevent such a slide could not in practice be made effective or, more fundamentally, because the ethical reasoning underlying the case for voluntary euthanasia also supports euthanasia without request.

1 The 'Practical Slope'

Are the criteria for voluntary euthanasia laid down by the Dutch courts and endorsed by the KNMG adequate to prevent instances of euthanasia which do not satisfy the criteria, especially the requirement of a free and well-considered request? It has been stressed by defenders of the Dutch criteria, such as Henk Rigter, Executive Director of the Health Council, that the guidelines for lawful euthanasia are both 'precisely defined' and 'strict'.[63] Are they?

(i) Identifying the criteria

Before deciding whether the criteria are precise and strict it is necessary accurately to identify them. The Supreme Court decided that necessity could operate as a defence to a charge under article 293 but omitted to state with any exactitude the criteria to be satisfied for the defence to apply. Even taking into account the decisions of lower courts, the criteria are not easy to determine. For example, Professor Leenen has written that each court decision has its own set of criteria, which creates 'much uncertainty'.[64]

(ii) 'Strict' and 'precise'?

Even if, say, Borst-Eilers's list of criteria were definitive there would still remain the question of the precision and strictness of those criteria. As for their supposed precision, Dutch jurists, such as Leenen, have remarked upon their vagueness. He defines euthanasia as a 'deliberate life-shortening act – including an omission to act – by a person other than the person concerned, at the request of the latter'.[65] He observes that other elements such as 'unbearable pain' are sometimes included but objects that they cannot form part of the definition – first, because they introduce judgements on which people disagree, and secondly because 'these elements cannot be delineated precisely'.[66] He continues that to include 'unbearable pain', whether physical or psychological, is to render the definition of euthanasia 'vague and useless' by stretching it to cover a broad range of human suffering.[67] Moreover, far from clarifying these inherent ambiguities the Supreme Court in the *Alkmaar* case appears to have compounded the problem by introducing such opaque concepts as 'death with dignity'.[68]

As for Rigter's claim that the criteria are 'strict', this too is difficult to sustain, not only because of their imprecision but also because of the absence of any satisfactory procedure, such as an effective independent check on the doctor's decision-making, to ensure that they are met.

Take, for example, the first criterion, that the request must come only from the patient and be 'entirely free and voluntary'.[69] What this means is not explained, and although the KNMG Guidelines state that the request must not be the result of pressure by others, they do not prevent either the doctor or nurse from mentioning euthanasia to the patient as an option or even strongly recommending it. Further, although the Guidelines provide that a request for euthanasia on the ground of being a nuisance to family should be an occasion to discuss alternative solutions, and that euthanasia is not to be administered because of problems which can be resolved in another way, they by no means rule out euthanasia in such a case.[70] Herbert Cohen, a GP who is one of Holland's leading practitioners of euthanasia, has said that he would be put in a very difficult position if a patient told him that he really felt a nuisance to his relatives because they wanted to enjoy his estate. Asked whether he would rule out euthanasia in such a case, Dr Cohen replied: 'I ... think in the end I wouldn't, because that kind of influence these children wanting the money now – is the same kind of power from the past that ... shaped us all. The same thing goes for religion ... education ... the kind of family he was raised in, all kinds of influences from the past that we can't put aside'.[71]

Even if the meaning of 'entirely free and voluntary' were clear, do doctors possess the expertise to determine whether a request fulfills this requirement? If they do, can the recommended procedure for ascertaining whether a request is free – the Guidelines merely recommend 'a' conversation[72], of unspecified length and content ensure that any such expertise is effectively deployed? Leenen, observing that a doctor can never know that a request is free and not the result of pressure from relatives, has commented: 'He does not know about emotional influence from the family ... He never knows about the annoyance which patients can be to the nursing staff sometimes. All these factors can ... be true'.[73]

Turning to the second criterion, that the request be 'well-considered, durable and persistent', the question again arises how all this is to be determined. How is the doctor to decide whether the request is the result of rational reflection or the influence of pain or drugs? As Kamisar has observed:

Undoubtedly, some euthanasia candidates will have their lucid moments. How they are to be distinguished from fellow-sufferers who do not, or how these instances are to be distinguished from others when the patient is exercising an irrational judgment is not an easy matter,

particularly when no psychiatrically-trained personnel assist in the assessment of the request.[74] He continues by asking whether, even if the mind of the 'pain-racked' patient is clear, it is not likely to be 'uncertain and variable'?[75]

The Guidelines merely state that one request is insufficient;[76] presumably two requests, even if made during the same consultation, would suffice. It is difficult to maintain that this is sufficient to meet Kamisar's point. Moreover, in assessing the practitioner's ability to ensure that a request is free, well-considered and durable, it is relevant to note that, on average, each GP in The Netherlands sees thirty patients per day in consultations lasting only seven to ten minutes.[77]

Doubts about whether the Guidelines can ensure that a request is well-considered and enduring have not been dispelled by a recent survey of GPs about euthanasia. The survey was carried out in 1990 by medical examiner van der Wal *et al.* It concluded that the interval between the first request for euthanasia and its performance was no more than a day in 13% of cases, no more than a week in another 35%, and no more than a fortnight in a further 17%, and that the interval between the last request for euthanasia and its performance was, in three out of five cases, no more than a day. The survey also found that in 22% of cases there was (contrary to the guidelines) only a single request and that in a further 30% of cases the interval between the first and last requests was between an hour and a week. Finally, in almost two-thirds of cases the request was purely oral.[78]

Further, Kamisar asks whether, even if the patient's request could be said to be clear and incontrovertible, other difficulties do not remain: 'Is this the kind of choice, assuming that it can be made in a fixed and rational manner, that we want to offer a gravely ill person? Will we not sweep up, in the process, some who are not really tired of life, but think others are tired of them ...?'[79]

Moving to the third criterion, 'intolerable suffering', the KNMG's Report declared that the concept is imprecise, not susceptible to objective verification, and can be caused by non-medical factors.[80] Moreover, van der Wal's survey found that although in 56% of official notifications 'intolerable suffering' was certified by doctors as the most important reason for euthanasia, only 42% of the patients had mentioned it as a reason and only 18% as their most important reason. 29% of patients gave 'senseless' suffering as their most important reason, and 24% 'fear/ anticipation of mental deterioration'.[81]

One argument against entrusting the euthanasia decision to the patient's doctor is that the doctor is fallible and that he may make errors in diagnosis or prognosis which could lead him to conclude, mistakenly, either that the patient's suffering is unbearable or that there is no means of palliation.[82] Here one may mention a report of the Health Council, published in 1987, on palliative care in The Netherlands. It concluded that 54% of cancer patients who were in pain suffered unnecessarily because doctors and nurses had insufficient understanding of the nature of the pain and the possibilities for its alleviation.[83] There is, moreover, the related argument that the doctor's objectivity can be swayed by emotional pressures; as Kamisar has commented: 'no man is immune to the fear, anxieties and frustrations engendered by the apparently helpless, hopeless patient'.[84]

Is the danger of fallibility, whether due to medical ignorance or emotional stresses, countered by the sixth criterion: consultation? It is questionable whether this criterion provides an effective safeguard against mis-interpretation and mis-application of the other criteria.

First, *if* consultation is a legal requirement at all, it may well only be required when there is doubt about the *medical* aspects of the case.[85] Now in a large proportion, if not the vast majority, of cases the doctor may well believe that there is no such doubt. Moreover, if consultation is not required when the diagnosis is clear, this suggests that when consultation is required, the requirement is satisfied if the second opinion is sought solely on the medical aspects of the case. The requirement of consultation is, then, hardly apt to allay concern about the difficulty of ensuring that the non-medical criteria are satisfied. Secondly, the consultation procedure recommended by the KNMG committee in 1984 has not been implemented. Nor has any court set out the form which consultation should take.[86] Thirdly, there is no requirement that the second doctor concur with the first doctor's interpretation of the criteria on which the second doctor is consulted or with their application to the patient in question. Further, the second doctor could adopt an interpretation of the criteria at least as relaxed as the first.

Even were consultation a universal practice it would, therefore, seem, of limited value as a check on the judgment or integrity of the first doctor. It is, moreover, far from universal. Van der Wal reports: 'One quarter of the general practitioners said they had not had *consultation* prior to euthanasia/assisted suicide ... More serious is the finding that 12% ... manifestly had no form of *discussion* with any other caregivers either'.[87] When consultation did occur the second opinion was in most cases a colleague rather than an independent doctor. Further, the second doctor already knew the patient in about 60% of cases and only put his opinion in writing in about a quarter of cases. Finally, fewer than half of the GPs consulted the patient's district nurse about his request for euthanasia.[88]

(iii) Empirical evidence

Another of Rigter's claims is that if a doctor were to press euthanasia on a patient 'this would surely be discovered, and the doctor would have to face charges of murder or manslaughter'.[89] Empirical evidence does not substantiate this claim.

Estimates of the number of cases of medical euthanasia in The Netherlands, which has a population of some 15 million and some 130 000 deaths per year, put the figure at at least 2000.[90] The survey by van der Wal estimates the annual number of cases of euthanasia and assisted suicide by general practitioners at 2000. However, the survey excludes cases in hospital, mainly on 'the assumption that the incidence of euthanasia and assisted suicide is greatest in the home situation'; it also excludes cases of the 'discontinuation of or failure to institute a treatment' at the patient's request.[91] Finally, in September 1991, a government committee, chaired by Attorney-General Remmelink, reported that its own survey of doctors revealed that in 1990 there were 2300 cases of voluntary euthanasia; 400 cases of assisted suicide; 1000 cases of life termination without an explicit request, and 15 975 cases in which it was the doctor's 'explicit' or 'secondary' intention to shorten life, either by administering pain-killing drugs (8100 cases) or by withholding or withdrawing treatment (7875 cases). In short, doctors admitted intending to shorten life in almost 20 000 cases.[92]

It is difficult to determine how many cases of euthanasia satisfy the legal criteria, not least because it appears that the overwhelming majority of cases are falsely certified as death by natural causes and are never reported and investigated. Reported cases for the years 1987–90 totalled 122; 181; 336 and 454 respectively.[93] Even if the lowest estimate of 2000 euthanasia cases per year were accurate, this would still mean underreporting by over 90% in 1988; over 80% in 1989, and over 70% in 1990. This fact places a large question mark against Rigter's claim that if the situation in The Netherlands is at all unique, 'it is perhaps in the wish of physicians to subject their actions to public scrutiny'.[94]

Borst-Eilers has stated that in unnotified cases there is no guarantee of propriety and that it is impossible to evaluate what the doctors have done.[95] Similarly, Mrs Tromp-Meesters, a spokesman for the DVES, has observed that under the present law 'there is no control', that the purpose of notification is merely statistical and that it is not an adequate safeguard against abuse.[96]

In short, notwithstanding the permissive character of the Dutch criteria for permissible euthanasia, there would appear to be no hard evidence that these criteria are being widely observed; on the contrary, the fact that, as just noted, the vast majority of deaths from euthanasia are illegally and incorrectly reported as natural deaths itself casts doubt on the lawfulness of much of the euthanasia which is being carried out. Moreover, it does not follow that the doctor who notifies the authorities has complied with the criteria; a doctor who has acted in breach of the law is no more likely to admit having done so in his report than a tax evader is likely to reveal his dishonesty on his tax return.

Moreover, whatever prospect there was of detecting abuse in a reported case has been reduced by the Minister of Justice's directive to prosecutors that they should order a police investigation only if the medical examiner's report reveals suspicious circumstances. One prosecutor regarded the directive (which, he revealed, had been introduced against the advice of the Chief Prosecutors) with dismay. He explained that the medical examiner does not have the necessary investigative expertise and conducts an inquiry which is 'just a chat between doctors and no inquiry at all'. The prosecutor added that the examiner's perfunctory certificate stating the cause of death was hardly of assistance in deciding whether the police should be asked to investigate. Under the previous system, he said, the prosecutor insisted on 'some hard facts' before deciding not to order an investigation. He continued that the directive had been welcomed by the medical profession because they saw it as an indication of the Minister's agreement with them that decisions about euthanasia should be made by doctors rather than by lawyers. 'So it can be', I asked, 'a little chat between the medical examiner and the doctor and that's how they would like it?' 'Yes, yes', he replied, adding that in the countryside there were some towns with only two or three doctors: 'What's the use', he said, 'of asking one of those two or three to judge the handling of a euthanasia case by the other one? How objective can that be? I don't see it'. He concluded that the new directive required prosecutors to lower their professional standards to what he regarded as below even the 'absolute minimum'.[97]

It is evident that the statistical evidence does nothing to refute allegations of non-voluntary and involuntary euthanasia which have been made by several Dutch experts. For example, Dr Fenigsen, a cardiologist at the Willem-Alexander Hospital, 's-Hertogenbosch, maintains that there is widespread public and professional support for euthanasia without request, as well as ample evidence of the practice.[98] Drawing on his own observations he declares: 'Doctors whose actions I observed, repeatedly tried to justify euthanasia by making reference to false data – citing a non-existent lung cancer, or a presumed, but never made, family request ...'.[99] He refers also to the work of experts such as Drs Hilhorst and van der Sluis. Dr Hilhorst, a sociologist who conducted empirical research in

Dutch hospitals, reported that doctors and nurses told him that requests for euthanasia came more frequently from the family than the patient and he concluded that both the family and the doctors and nurses often pressured the patient to request euthanasia.[100] Dr van der Sluis, a dermatologist involved with the treatment of AIDS patients, states that non-voluntary and involuntary euthanasia are common and openly defended in medical journals.[101]

Moreover, in a survey by medical lawyer Professor van Wijmen, 123 doctors, or 41% of the respondents, admitted that they had performed euthanasia without the patient's request. 88 had done so in 1–4 cases; 24 in 5–10 cases; 4 in 11–15 cases; and 7 in more than 15 cases.[102]

Further, the Remmelink Committee reported that in 1000 cases in 1990, life was terminated without an explicit request from the patient and that in 13 691 cases the doctor's 'explicit' or 'secondary' intention was to shorten life without request, either by withholding or withdrawing treatment (8750 cases) or by administering pain-killing drugs (4941 cases). In short, doctors intended to shorten life without request in some 15 000 cases.[103]

Other evidence of euthanasia without request is provided by a number of criminal prosecutions. Professor Sluyters, a medical lawyer, mentions one case in 1985 involving a doctor who was convicted of killing several patients in a nursing home in The Hague and who was sentenced to one year's imprisonment; his conviction was quashed because the police had improperly seized incriminating documents and he was awarded 300 000 guilders (approximately £85 000) compensation for the six months he had already spent in prison. Sluyters also refers to cases in which nurses were convicted of killing handicapped children. Although expressing his support for 'the Dutch solution of restrained liberalisation' of the law relating to euthanasia, he concedes: 'In the Netherlands we have seen some cases in the courts in recent years which could perhaps be illustrating the adverse consequences of the liberalisation of euthanasia'.[104] Again, Borst-Eilers has commented that, although she did not believe that voluntary euthanasia led logically to involuntary euthanasia, 'if I am honest I must admit that I cannot judge whether the fact that euthanasia is openly talked about does not bring about a kind of feeling that it's something that you are allowed to do' and that this might have influenced the doctor and nurses in the above cases to perform euthanasia without request.[105]

In sum, the legal and medical criteria for euthanasia would not appear to constitute an effective safeguard against the practice of non-voluntary and involuntary euthanasia. Moreover, the evidence of critics of the Dutch euthanasia experience, such as Fenigsen and van der Sluis, suggests that what the criteria are sufficiently loose to permit is indeed taking place. There is, moreover, a dearth of evidence to support contrary claims that the criteria are being generally observed; as the KNMG indicated in its report, the failure of doctors to notify would mean the legality and propriety of what was happening in practice would be 'absolutely unverifiable'.[106]

2 The 'logical slope'

Even if doubts about the criteria for lawful euthanasia were dispelled, there would remain the question whether these criteria state necessary as opposed to merely sufficient conditions for lawful euthanasia. Is the legal reasoning of the Supreme Court and the ethical reasoning of the Dutch proponents of euthanasia based upon a principle which entails that some or even all of the existing criteria are superfluous?

(i) The legal slope

In fact, in the *Alkmaar* case, the Supreme Court did not lay down a list of necessary criteria for lawful euthanasia; its judgment was framed in more general terms. It held that necessity was available as a defence to euthanasia and that in determining the availability of the defence in a given case, a crucial question was whether there was a situation of necessity according to 'responsible medical opinion', tested by 'prevailing standards of medical ethics'.[107]

This suggests that the existence of necessity in a given case is to be determined primarily by criteria fashioned by the medical profession rather than by the courts. Commenting on the case Sutorious observes that according to the Supreme Court 'the primary judgment should remain with the medical discipline, the second judgment is a legal one and should rest with society' and he adds that in his opinion the court 'wishes to have euthanasia problems solved where they arise, notably in the medical discipline'.[108]

However, it is doubtful whether there is a consensus within the profession about the conditions justifying euthanasia and in the absence of an agreed set of criteria there will only be disparate bodies of medical opinion. Medical opinion is often divided over purely technical matters such as diagnosis and treatment, a fact recognised by the common law's test for medical negligence which refuses to hold a doctor negligent merely because he acted in accordance with one responsible body of medical opinion rather than another.[109] Medical opinion is likely to be at least as split over an ethical issue such as euthanasia. Presumably, a doctor performing euthanasia will not incur criminal liability if he acts in accordance with a body of medical opinion. But, does this not render the current criteria essentially provisional? Moreover, how is a court in determining what amounts to a 'responsible medical opinion' to select expert witnesses and how is it to proceed if they disagree?

The centrality attached by the Supreme Court to medical opinion has attracted the criticism of a number of Dutch jurists. Feber concludes that the court's decision to cede so much influence to medical opinion leaves insufficient room for the judge to arrive at an independent decision.[110] Leenen has observed: 'By referring to medical ethics the Supreme Court left the problem of the criteria for the acceptability of euthanasia on request in essence unsolved. Moreover, the reference is useless because of the ... disagreement within the medical profession upon ethics'.[111]

However, even if doctors were unanimous about the appropriate criteria, there would still be several weighty objections to the Supreme Court's reasoning. First, if the Court is effectively entrusting the determination of the lawfulness of euthanasia to the medical profession, does this not amount to an abdication of judicial responsibility? Mulder argues that the legal boundaries of euthanasia should be made by the judiciary as representatives of society and not by the medical profession.[112]

Secondly, are doctors, whose training is in medicine, not ethics or law, competent to determine when, if ever, euthanasia is justifiable?

Thirdly, are the existing criteria, which are presumably in line with 'reasonable' medical opinion, consistent with the principles informing Dutch criminal law, particularly that, instantiated in article 293, which requires the protection of human life? Mulder points out that whereas an act intended to alleviate the suffering of a dying patient which has the foreseen consequence of accelerating the death of the patient has been permitted by Dutch law, to allow the intentional killing of a patient to alleviate suffering is a new departure.[113]

Fourthly, the decisions of the Court contain no adequate analysis of the doctor's duty to the patient nor reason why the alleviation of suffering should override the clear terms of article 293. The decisions are all the more remarkable when it is recalled that the very terms of the article emphasise that the victim's earnest request, let alone consent, is no defence to a charge of homicide. Sluyters has written that article 293 was enacted primarily 'to leave no doubt that the killing of a person is unlawful even if that person desires death'.[114] Moreover, the Explanatory Memorandum to article 293 explains that, although one who takes the life of another at his request should be punished 'considerably less severely than those guilty of plain murder', the victim's consent 'cannot abolish the criminality of taking someone's life'. It continues: 'the law so to speak no longer punishes the assault on the life of a particular person, but rather the violation of the respect due to human life in general – irrespective of the offender's motive. The criminal offence against life remains, the assault against the person expires'.[115] Again, Mulder, having noted that life has value to the community as well as to the individual, observes that it is 'certain that the Lawgiver considered life worth protecting, even when it no longer has any value to the individual'.[116]

Neither the letter nor the spirit of the Code, then, appears to give any support to the Supreme Court's decision that a defence to a charge under article 293 is implicit in article 40. Indeed, had the legislature intended to provide a defence to article 293 it could have done so expressly. There seems no evidence or reason to doubt that the legislature decided that the protection of life took priority over the autonomy of the individual or the alleviation of suffering. By holding that a doctor may choose to kill in order to relieve suffering, the Court inverted (without any show of juridically sufficient reason) the legislature's ordering of values.

But perhaps the legislature did not foresee the acute suffering which can be imposed on patients by, or as a side effect of, modern medical technology? Perhaps the prohibition in article 293 is outdated and could not have been intended to apply in contemporary Holland? But, in 1891 as today, the legislature must have been well aware that people typically seek euthanasia precisely to avoid suffering. There is no reason to think that the legislature was willing to allow the alleviation of even 'unbearable' suffering to take priority over the protection of life, or that the suffering experienced today is greater than when article 293 was enacted. As Driesse observes:

Despite the fact that people were deeply persuaded that life could bring much and serious suffering, and despite the fact that in those days there were also people who requested death, the lawgiver in Article 293 ... did not abrogate punishment.[117]

Moreover, it would be reasonable to conclude that, with modern palliative care, the suffering which leads people to request euthanasia is substantially less today than it was when article 293 was enacted. Driesse concludes:

To change this article ... by declaring killing on request, or alternatively rendering assistance in self-killing, to be non-punishable in certain instances, is not the adaptation of an obsolete regulation which is required by changed circumstances. It is the concretization of a fundamental change of attitude in regard to the inviolability of the human individual and of respect for human life.[118]

To all this one must add that the legal position thus reached in 1984 would be rendered all the more far-reaching if the Supreme Court were clearly to hold that the defence of duress in euthanasia cases could extend to 'mental duress' *suffered by the defendant healthcare professional*. Mulder has commented that the courts should not be too eager to allow this type of defence as it paves the way to 'euthanasia-like' acts by other experts, especially nursing personnel.[119] But one must go further: to allow this defence of mental duress is already, in principle, to have accepted *in*voluntary euthanasia, since the request or the consent of the person killed is quite irrelevant within the framework of such a defence.

(ii) The ethical slope

The main argument advanced in The Netherlands for legalising voluntary euthanasia has been that it respects the individual's right to self-determination. Leenen, for example, argues that interference with that right can only be justified if it is to protect essential social values, which is not the case where patients suffering unbearably at the end of their lives request euthanasia when no alternatives exist. He adds: 'Not allowing people euthanasia would come down to forcing them to suffer against their will, which would be cruel and a negation of their human rights and dignity'.[120] Echoing other proponents of legalisation,[121] he observes that modern medicine has contributed to the prolongation of suffering and the 'disfigurement of dying'[122] and he advances arguments in favour of the *statutory* legalisation of euthanasia such as the need to protect self-determination by ensuring that euthanasia is only carried out at the free, explicit and serious request of the patient, and the need to guarantee that doctors, who may be influenced by emotion, exercise great care in making the decision. He points to the legislative proposals of the State Commission on Euthanasia which reported in 1985 and which recommended that article 293 be amended to provide that it would not be unlawful to terminate the life of another at his express and serious request when he was in an 'untenable situation without any prospects' and when the termination was carried out by a doctor 'within the framework of careful medical practice'.[123]

Dutch advocates of legalisation take pains to stress that they support *voluntary* euthanasia but oppose *in*voluntary euthanasia. Their position on *non*-voluntary euthanasia is often obscure, largely because of a tendency to confine discussion to the voluntary type. This is often effected by adopting Leenen's definition of euthanasia as *voluntary* euthanasia[124] and declining to regard as euthanasia the termination of life without the patient's request.

Notwithstanding the difficulty of ascertaining their complete ethical position, there is some evidence that many of the Dutch proponents of euthanasia in fact regard the existing criteria for legal euthanasia as sufficient but by no means morally necessary conditions. For example, in relation to the criterion of 'unbearable suffering', Tromp-Meesters has stated that the DVES would ideally like the law to allow anyone to ask their doctor for euthanasia even in the absence of such suffering: 'If you can convince your doctor that you have good reasons to want to die, the doctor should feel free to help you'.[125] *She* felt that ideally it would be like ancient Rome where (she says) once a year citizens could ask to be put to death.[126]

Again, there is widespread support for euthanasia even though the patient is incompetent. The State Commission, for example, recommended that 'the intentional termination of the life of a person unable to express his or her will should not be an offence provided this is performed by a physician in the context of careful medical procedure in respect of a patient who, according to the current state of medical knowledge, has irreversibly lost consciousness, and provided also that treatment has been suspended as pointless'.[127]

Further, the KNMG Report in 1984 did not condemn euthanasia without request but simply confined itself, for the time being, to euthanasia for those who were capable of expressing their will. Indeed, it did not even address the ethics of euthanasia but merely observed that euthanasia was practised and that in a pluralistic society views on the subject would always differ.[128] This approach could, of course, also be used to approve euthanasia without request. Indeed, in 1988 a KNMG working party condoned euthanasia for malformed infants,[129] concluding that in certain situations the doctor ought to terminate life.[130] In 1991, a KNMG committee considering 'Life-Ending Treatment of Incompetent Patients' advocated the killing of patients in persistent coma.[131]

Finally, leading proponents of euthanasia have occasionally expressed support for euthanasia without request. Asked whether he saw any moral distinction between removing artificial feeding from a comatose patient and actively killing him, Dr Admiraal replied: 'No, I should kill the patient as well ... In a coma there is no ... suffering ... and there is no consciousness so there is no ... reason to stop life immediately but I should do [so] and not wait for the starving of that patient for the next weeks. Oh no, I should say if I made the decision to stop tube-feeding, I should give active euthanasia ...'. He added that it was the same situation with a neonate: 'You can't speak about voluntary euthanasia, it's only the parents asking for ... the judgement of the doctors and you are just killing that baby'. Asked whether there was anything wrong with that, he replied that he did not think so.[132]

The above considerations suggest that a substantial number of the most prominent Dutch advocates of voluntary euthanasia in fact support non-voluntary euthanasia. They may, moreover, be logically committed to this position, for the basis of their case for voluntary euthanasia, namely, respect for self-determination, may well be thought to provide little or no ground for judging wrongful the euthanatising of those who do not possess autonomy, whether because they are infants, senile adults, mentally handicapped, or comatose. The widespread condonation of euthanasia in the case of the comatose is particularly revealing, for it undermines the need for either a request or for suffering (whether unbearable or not) and suggests that the right to self-determination is, notwithstanding the emphasis commonly placed upon it, an incomplete explanation of the case for euthanasia which is advanced in The Netherlands. The case would appear fundamentally to rest on the principle that lives which fall below a certain 'quality' are not worth living. This principle has evidently been openly adopted by some of the leading Dutch exponents of euthanasia. For example, Professor van der Meer, former Head of Internal Medicine at the Free University of Amsterdam, has written that it is obvious that the 'quality of life' of a person rendered permanently comatose has fallen 'below the minimum'.[133]

Of course, if the Dutch case for voluntary euthanasia is, as it would appear to be, based on the principle that certain lives are not worth living, then it raises the questions whether this principle is defensible and whether it does not logically permit non-voluntary and even involuntary euthanasia. One of the unfortunate consequences of the emphasis in the Dutch euthanasia debate on the right of self-determination has been that these important questions have not received the attention they deserve. They have, however, been addressed by opponents of legalisation, notably Kamisar. He concludes that there is a real danger of sliding down the 'slippery slope', first because it has already taken place this century and started with the acceptance of the attitude that there is such a thing as a life not worth living[134] and secondly because, as he demonstrates, many supporters of voluntary euthanasia have historically shared this attitude.[135] He argues, moreover, that reasons which have been advanced by proponents of voluntary euthanasia for not extending euthanasia to the senile and the defective are much more tentative and unpersuasive than the arguments they deploy for legalising euthanasia in the first place.[136]

Conclusion

The significance of the Dutch euthanasia experience for law, medicine and social policy in other countries is considerable, not least in respect of the support it lends to the 'slippery slope' argument. Some have argued that the danger of a slide into non-voluntary and involuntary euthanasia would be reduced if the criteria were statutory. It will be recalled that Leenen listed arguments in favour of legislation, such as the need to ensure that euthanasia was only performed at the patient's request.[137] He omits, however, to explain *how* legislation would provide more effective safeguards against abuse. Moreover, as medical lawyer Professor Gevers has cautioned: 'It is impossible to delineate precisely the situations in which euthanasia should be allowed; therefore, a new law cannot add very much to what has already been developed by the courts, and will only partially reduce legal uncertainty'.[138] Further, the legislative proposals contained in the report of the State Commission on Euthanasia are, as Leenen himself has observed,[139] essentially the same as those developed by the courts. Indeed, it is arguable that the central criterion proposed by the Commission, an 'untenable situation' with no prospect of improvement[140], is even looser than the existing criterion of unbearable suffering which cannot be alleviated.

It could, of course, be argued that although euthanasia without request may be practised in The Netherlands, it is also carried out in jurisdictions where euthanasia is unlawful, such as the UK, and that the legalisation of voluntary euthanasia helps prevent the carrying out of euthanasia without request. As a spokesman for the KNMG put it, there is a choice between on the one hand prohibiting euthanasia and not knowing how often it is carried out and, on the other hand, legalising it and knowing how most of it is carried out. The KNMG, he explained, wanted it to be controlled, and if it were prohibited, it could not be controlled.[141] But it is clear from the evidence set out in Part III 1 (iii) above that all that is known with certainty in The Netherlands is that euthanasia is being practised on a scale vastly exceeding the 'known' (truthfully reported and recorded) cases. There is little sense in which it can be said, in any of its forms, to be under control. As Leenen has observed, there is an 'almost total lack of control on the administration of euthanasia'[142] and 'the present legal situation makes any adequate control of the practice of euthanasia virtually impossible'.[143]

The lack of any effective control over the practice of euthanasia in Holland has recently been confirmed by Dr Carlos Gomez. The extent to which the Dutch control euthanasia is the central concern of his book *Regulating Death: Euthanasia and the Case of the Netherlands*[144] which documents Dr Gomez's empirical investigation of this question.

He begins by asking: 'How will we assure ourselves that the weak, the demented, the vulnerable, the stigmatized – those incapable of consent or dissent – [will] not become the unwilling subjects of such a practice?'[145] He observes that it is commonly agreed that prosecutors review only a small minority of cases and he concludes that, therefore, the 'formal, juridical level' of the Dutch regulatory system is 'routinely bypassed'.[146] As for the 'informal' regulatory criteria laid down by the KNMG, Gomez concludes: 'not only are they not enforced, they are probably unenforceable'.[147] He adds that the role of regulated and regulator has fallen to doctors with the tacit consent of Dutch society and that this bespeaks not only a remarkable trust in the medical profession but also an 'almost cavalier attitude toward those – however many or few their numbers – who cannot challenge a decision to have euthanasia performed upon them'.[148] He concludes that 'on the core issues of the controversy – how to control the practice, how to keep it from being used on those who do not want it, how to provide for public accountability – the Dutch response has been, to date, inadequate'.[149]

Notes

1 This research was generously funded by the British Academy whose support I gratefully acknowledge. I also appreciate supplementary sums provided by the Dutch Ministry of Education and by my Department. Thanks are also due to the following for their invaluable assistance: Dr Maurice de Wachter, Hub Zwart and Ingrid Ravenschlag of the Instituut voor Gezondheidsethiek, Maastricht; Therese te Braake, Nicole de Bijl (of the Department of Health Law) and Jurgen Worestshofer, Job Cohen and Louise Rayar (of the Department of Law) at the State University of Limburg; Henk Jochemsen of the Lindeboom Instituut, Ede; Dr Martens, of the Royal Dutch Medical Association (KNMG); Drs Admiraal, Cohen, van der Meer and Gunning; Mrs Tromp-Meesters and Professor Dupuis of the Dutch Voluntary Euthanasia Society (DVES); Eugene Sutorius, Counsel to the Society; Mrs Borst-Eilers, Vice-President of the Dutch Health Council; H J J Leenen, Emeritus Professor of Social Medicine and Health Law at the University of

Amsterdam; two public prosecutors, one in Rotterdam, the other in
Alkmaar; Attorney-General Remmelink and his Secretary Mr den Hartog
Jager; Mr Stryards and Mr Kors, legal advisers at the Ministry of Justice,
and Professor J M Finnis of University College, Oxford, who commented on
an earlier draft of this paper.

Unless the contrary is apparent, all translations are by Hub Zwart, to
whom I owe a special debt of thanks. All references to 'interviews' refer to
interviews I conducted between July 1989 and December 1991. Unless
attributed to another, the views expressed in this paper are mine and I
remain solely responsible for the accuracy of the paper.

2 Quotations from the Penal Code are taken from an unpublished translation
of the Code by Louise Rayar.

3 *Ibid.*

4 B Sluyters, 'Euthanasia in The Netherlands' (1989) 57(1) *Medico-Legal
Journal* 34, 35.

5 *Ibid.*

6 Rayar, *op. cit* n2, *supra.*

7 Jurgen Woretshofer, 'Current Court Decisions and Legislation on
Euthanasia in The Netherlands' (pages 25–51 of an unpublished manuscript
on euthanasia) 26. (Page references correspond to those in the manuscript.)
Articles 293 and 294 were added to the Penal Code in 1891. H J J Leenen,
'Euthanasia in the Netherlands' in Peter Byrne (ed) *Medicine, Medical Ethics
and the Value of Life* (1990) 10.

8 See generally H J J Leenen, 'Euthanasia, assistance to suicide and the law:
developments in the Netherlands' (1987) 8 *Health Policy* 197, 200–2; *op. cit.*
n7, *supra*, 4–6.

The pyramidal structure of the criminal court system rises from the
sixty-two Cantonal Courts, which deal with minor offences, through the
nineteen District Courts, each covering three or four cantons, to the five
Courts of Appeal, each of which covers three or four districts. At the apex is
the Supreme Court, which is concerned solely with questions of law. See
Peter Zisser, 'Euthanasia and the Right to Die: Holland and the United
States face the Dilemma' (1988) 9 *New York Law School Journal of
International and Comparative Law* 361, 365n53.

9 *Nederlandse Jurisprudentie* (hereafter *NJ*) (1985) No 106.

10 J K M Gevers, 'Legal Developments concerning active Euthanasia on
Request in The Netherlands' (1987) 1 *Bioethics* 156, 159. The case report
reads as follows:

At the trial . . . counsel for the accused appealed to necessity [*overmacht*] in
the sense that the accused found himself confronted by a "conflict of
duties, in which he came to a right choice in a well-considered manner".
This appeal to a conflict of duties, which should be distinguished from the
accused's appeal to necessity in the sense of constraint of conscience
[*gewetensdrang*], can hardly be interpreted otherwise than as an appeal to
emergency [*noodtoestand*], which amounts to the accused carefully
weighing the duties and interests which faced each other in this case,
especially in accordance with the norms of medical ethics and with the
expertise which he, as a physician, can be expected to possess; and making
a decision which – considered objectively and in view of the special
circumstances in this case – was justified.'   (*NJ* (1985) No 106, 451 at 452)
The report continues (at 452–3) that the Court of Appeal had properly
rejected the defence of 'constraint of conscience' but that its rejection of the

defence of 'emergency' was unsound as it failed to take into account the condition of Mrs B. and the fact that the accused in his 'competent judgement as a physician' felt that she experienced each day of life as 'a heavy burden under which she suffered unbearably'. In view of this, the Supreme Court continued (at 453):

> further clarification is needed as to why the Court of Appeal ... still comes to the judgement that it "has not become sufficiently plausible" that the suffering of B. at the very moment the accused terminated her life ... should be considered so unbearable that the accused in fairness had no other choice than to spare her this suffering by means of euthanasia ... Rather it should have gone without saying that the Appeal Court, after having determined the facts and circumstances ... [relating to B's condition], would have further investigated whether, according to well-considered medical judgement and in accordance with medico-ethical norms [*nader zou hebben onderzocht of naar verantwoord medisch inzicht, getoetst aan in de medische ethiek geldende normen*], it was a matter of emergency as claimed by the accused.

11 Rayar, *op. cit.* n2, *supra*.
12 Woretshofer, *op. cit.* n7, *supra*, 38.
13 'The High Court of the Hague, Case No. 79065, October 21, 1986; (edited and translated by Barry A Bostrom and Walter Lagerwey) (1988) 3 *Issues in Law & Medicine* 445, 448. Bostrom and Lagerwey attribute this and other passages from the 'Note', appended to the report of the case, to A.-G. Remmelink. As the initials 'G.E.M.' at the end of the Note indicate, however, it is in fact by Mulder.
14 *NJ* (1985) No 106 451 at 453 (translated by Gevers, *op. cit.* n10, *supra*, 159–60).
15 Abstract (prepared from a translation and summary by Dr Walter Lagerwey) of H R G Feber, 'De wederwaardigheden van artikel 293 van het Wetboek van Strafrecht vanaf 1981 tot heden' ('The Vicissitudes of article 293 of the Penal Code from 1981 to the Present') in GA van der Wal, ed, *Euthanasie: Knelpunten in Een Discussie* ('*Euthanasia: Bottlenecks in a Discussion*') (1987) 54–81' in (1988) 3 *Issues in Law & Medicine* 455, 458. (Emphasis in original.)
16 *NJ* (1987) No 608.
17 Feber, *op. cit.* n15, *supra*, 462.
18 *Ibid.*
19 *Ibid*, 463–4.
20 *NJ* (1987) No 607.
21 See *op. cit.* n13, *supra*, 445.
22 *Ibid*, 445–6. (Emphasis in translation.) The Court held: 'The Court of Appeal should have considered whether the accused, as she arrived at her decision and proceeded to execute it, acted in emergency [*noodtoestand*] or psychological compulsion [*psychische overmacht*]'. *NJ* (1987) No 607 at 2124. In his 'Note' appended to the report of the case, Mulder observes that two differences strike him between the Supreme Court decisions of 1984 and 1986. One is that in the 1984 case the accused was the patient's physician whereas in the 1986 case she was not. The other is that in the latter decision, the Court 'provides an appeal to psychological compulsion [*psychische overmacht*] a chance of success'. *NJ* (1987) No 607 at 2129.
23 *Op. cit.* n13, *supra*, 446.
24 Because, says, Leenen, she did not consult another doctor. *op. cit.* n8, *supra*,

202. A further appeal to the Supreme Court was dismissed *NJ* (1989)
No 391. Attorney-General Remmelink informed me that in the light of this
case, psychological compulsion is only a 'theoretical' defence especially for
doctors, whom the courts expect to act in a professional manner (Interview,
26 November, 1991).

25 E Borst-Eilers, 'The Status of Physician-Administered Active Euthanasia in
The Netherlands' (Unpublished paper delivered at the Second International
Conference on Health Law and Ethics, London, July 1989) 3. See also
Leenen, *op. cit.* n8, *supra* 200; Sluyters, *op. cit.*, n4, *supra*, 41; Gevers, *op. cit.*
n10, *supra*, 158.

26 Interview, 10 July 1989. In the *Alkmaar* case the Appeal Court ruled that
although the accused had consulted his assistant and Mrs B.'s son, their
opinions were insufficiently independent. The Supreme Court held that this
did not prevent the euthanatising of Mrs B. from being an act in 'emergency'
according to 'objective medical judgement' *NJ* (1985) No 106 451 at 453.
Again, A N A Josephus Jitta, a public prosecutor, has written that the
requirement of a second opinion was 'abandoned once by the Dutch
Supreme Court in 1987' when it dismissed the case against a doctor who had
been prosecuted solely because he had not consulted. 'The Right to
Euthanasia in the Terminal Period' in *The Right to Self-Determination:
Proceedings of the 8th World Conference of the International Federation of
Right to Die Societies* (1990) 47, 48.

27 'Court of the Hague (Penal Chamber) April 2, 1987', (edited and translated
by Barry A. Bostrom and Walter Lagerwey) (1988) 3 *Issues in Law &
Medicine* 451.

28 *Ibid*, 452. Affirmed, *NJ* (1988) No 811.

29 Feber, *op. cit.* n15, *supra*, 462. The Prosecutor had sought the advice of the
KNMG about the defence of necessity and, when the Association replied
that euthanasia was permissible if the patient was suffering unbearably and
had made a free and well-considered request, had moved for the prosecution
to be dismissed. *Ibid*, 461.

30 Gevers, *op. cit.* n10, *supra*, 158.

31 'Standpunt inzake euthanasie' (Position on euthanasia) (1984) 39 *Medisch
Contact* 990. Quotations from the Report are taken from an unpublished
translation by the KNMG entitled 'Vision on Euthanasia' (hereafter
'Vision'). The translated version states that it has undated the Report on a
few points to take account of developments in law, politics and within the
KNMG until the end of 1986.

32 *Op. cit.* n25, *supra*, 3.

33 In collaboration with the National Association of Nurses.

34 'Guidelines for Euthanasia' (translated by Lagerwey) (1988) 3 *Issues in Law
& Medicine* 429. Hereafter 'Guidelines'.

35 Vision, 8–11.

36 Guidelines, 431–3.

37 Vision, 8.

38 *Ibid*, 9.

39 Guidelines, 431.

40 Vision, 9.

41 Guidelines, 432.

42 Vision, 9.

43 *Ibid*, 10.

44 Guidelines, 432.

45 Vision, 10.
46 *Ibid.*
47 *Ibid*, 11.
48 *Ibid.*
49 See text at n30.
50 Vision, 12.
51 *Ibid.*
52 *Ibid*, 12–13.
53 *Ibid*, 14.
54 Borst-Eilers, *op. cit.* n25, *supra*, 5.
55 *Ibid.*
56 *Ibid.*
57 Interview with public prosecutor, Alkmaar, 7 December 1990.
58 Leenen, *op. cit.* n8, *supra*, 200.
59 Interview with public prosecutor, Rotterdam, 31 July 1989.
60 Working Party of the Church of England's Board for Social Responsibility, *On Dying Well: An Anglican Contribution to the Debate on Euthanasia* (1975), 62.
61 Law Reform Commission of Canada, *Euthanasia, Aiding Suicide and Cessation of Treatment* (Report 20; 1983) 18.
62 *Euthanasia:Report of the Working Party to review the British Medical Associations' guidance on euthanasia* (1988) 4; 6; 31; 59.
63 Henk Rigter, 'Euthanasia in The Netherlands: Distinguishing Facts from Fiction' (1989) 19(1) *Hastings Center Report* 31.
64 H J J Leenen, 'Dying with Dignity: Developments in the Field of Euthanasia in the Netherlands' (1989) 8 *Medicine and Law* 517, 523. See also M A M de Wachter, 'Active Euthanasia in the Netherlands' (1989) 262 *Journal of the American Medical Association* 3316, 3317.
65 H J J Leenen, 'The Definition of Euthanasia' (1984) 3 *Medicine and Law* 333, 334.
66 *Ibid.*
67 *Ibid.*
68 See text at n14.
69 See text at n25.
70 Guidelines, 432.
71 Interview, 26 July 1989. 'Not wanting to be a (continued) burden on family/surroundings' was mentioned by 22% of patients in van der Wal's survey as a reason for requesting euthanasia. *Op. cit.* n78, *infra*, 214 Table 5.
72 See text at n39.
73 Interview, 24 July 1989.
74 Yale Kamisar, 'Some Non-Religious Views against Proposed "Mercy-Killing" Legislation' (1958) 42 *Minnesota Law Review* 969, in Dennis J. Horan and David Mall (eds), *Death, Dying and Euthanasia* (1980) 406, 425.
75 *Ibid.*
76 Guidelines, 432.
77 Interview, Dr Martens, 24 July 1989.
78 G van der Wall *et al.*, 'Euthanasie en hulp bij zelfdoding' (Euthanasia and Assisted Suicide) (1991) 56(7) *Medisch Contact* 211, 212–14 Tables 2, 3, 4, & 7. This paper is the third of four published in the KNMG journal in February 1991 which contain the methodology and results of van der Wal's survey. The papers have been translated by the Hemlock Society. Quotations

are taken from this unpublished translation; page references are to the journal.

79 *Op. cit.* n74, *supra*, 427.
80 Vision, 10–11.
81 Van der Wal, *op. cit.* n78, *supra*, 214 Table 5.
82 See generally Kamisar, *op. cit.* 74, *supra*, 430–5.
83 Interview, Gunning, 2 August 1989. Dr P. Sluis, a founder in 1987 of the Dutch Hospice Movement, has observed that palliative care is not very good in The Netherlands: 'The Dutch Hospice Movement', in *op. cit.* n26, *supra*, 97, 103.
84 *Op. cit*, n74, *supra*, 429.
85 See text at n26.
86 This was stated by Sutorius in an interview on 10 July 1989. There is, indeed, no legal requirement that the second doctor should even see the patient and a public prosecutor told me that it has by no means been a universal practice for the second doctor to see the patient. Interview, Rotterdam, 31 July 1989.
87 G van der Wal *et al.*, 'Toetsing in geval van euthanasie of hulp bij zelfdoding' (Verification in Euthanasia or Assisted Suicide) (1991) 46(8) *Medisch Contact* 237, 239. (Emphasis in original.)
88 *Ibid*, 240.
89 Henk Rigter *et al.*, 'Euthanasia across the North Sea' (1988) 297 *British Medical Journal* 1593, 1594.
90 See de Wachter, *op. cit.* n64, *supra*, 3316. Jitta has written that according to the estimate of the Central Medical Inspection of National Health, euthanasia is performed at least 6000 times per year in general practice and that if hospitals and nursing homes are added, the total is 10 000–12 000 cases: quoted in C I Dessaur and C J C Rutenfrans, 'The Present Day Practice of Euthanasia' (1988) 3 *Issues in Law & Medicine* 399, 400.
91 G van der Wal *et al.* 'Euthanasie en hulp bij zelfdoding door huisartsen' (Euthanasia and Assisted Suicide by GPs) (1991) 46(6) *Medisch Contact* 171. See also *ibid*, 174–6. The study's assumption would appear to require justification for, as Admiraal informed me, only some 30% of deaths occur at home. Interview, 27 July 1989.
92 Richard Fenigsen, 'The Netherlands: First Reactions to the Report of the Committee on Euthanasia' (1991) (Unpublished summary of *Medische beslissingen rond het levenseinde: Rapport van de Commissie onderzoek medische praktijk inzake euthanasie* (Sdu Uitgeverij Plantijnstraat, 's-Gravenhage, 1991) 1–2. See also Paul J van der Maas *et al.*, 'Euthanasia and other medical decisions concerning the end of life' (1991) 338 *Lancet* 669; K F Gunning, *ibid.*, 1010. See also Richard Fenigsen, 'The Report of the Dutch Governmental Committee on Euthanasia' (1991) *Issues in Law & Medicine* 339.
93 Personal communication from Stryards, 6 September 1991, citing *Javerslaag Openbaar Ministerie 1990* (1991) 59.
94 *Op. cit.* n63, *supra*, 32. Remmelink reported that three-quarters of GPs and almost two thirds of specialists who carried out euthanasia or assisted suicide in 1990 had falsely certified death by natural causes. Fenigsen, *op. cit.* n92, *supra*, 343. Almost half of the GPs in van der Wal's study had made no record of their last euthanasia case and, of those who had, fewer than half had done so in the form of a separate record. *op. cit.* n87, *supra*, 240. His general conclusion is that 'a substantial proportion of general practitioners is not (yet) operating in accordance with current procedural precautionary requirements'. *ibid*, 241.

95 Interview, 1 August 1989.
96 Interview, 11 July 1989.
97 Interview, public prosecutor, Alkmaar, 7 December 1990.
98 'A Case against Dutch Euthanasia' (1989) 19(1) *Hastings Centre Report* 22, 25.
99 *Ibid*, 30. See also Richard Fenigsen 'Euthanasia in the Netherlands' (1990) 6, *Issues in Law & Medicine* 229, 235–242.
100 Quoted in Barry A Bostrom, 'Euthanasia in the Netherlands: A Model for the United States? (1989) 4 *Issues in Law & Medicine* 467, 477.
101 I van der Sluis, 'The Practice of Euthanasia in the Netherlands' (1989) 4 *Issues in Law & Medicine* 455, 463.
102 F C B van Wijmen, *Artsen en het Zelfgekozen Levenseinde* (*Doctors and the Self-Chosen Termination of Life*) (1989) 24, Table 18. Van Wijmen observes that as cases of 'pseudo-euthanasia' (such as the withdrawal of futile treatment) were expressly excluded in the question, the answers are 'amazing'. *Ibid*. Again, in their book on euthanasia published in 1986, Professor Dessaur and Dr Rutenfrans, of the Criminology Department at the University of Nijmegen maintain that genuinely voluntary euthanasia amounts to no more than 10% of the 6000–12 000 cases per year. *Op. cit.* n90, *supra*, 401–2.
103 Fenigsen, *op. cit.* n92, *supra*, 341.
104 Sluyters, *op. cit.* n4, *supra*, 42. See also Ph. Schepens, 'Euthanasia: Our Own Future?' (1988) 3 *Issues in Law & Medicine* 371, 376–7; Fenigsen, *op. cit.* n98, *supra*, 25.
105 Interview, 1 August 1989.
106 Vision, 14.
107 See text at n10.
108 Eugene Ph R Sutorius, 'A Mild Death for Paragraph 293 of the Netherlands Criminal Code?' (Unpublished paper, 1986), 7.
109 *Bolam v. Friern Hospital Management Committee* [1957] 1 WLR 582.
110 *Op cit.* n15, *supra*, 458.
111 *Op cit.* n8, *supra*, 201.
112 *Op. cit.* n13, *supra*, 449.
113 *Ibid*, 446. Dr Admiraal has stated that he sees no moral difference between intentionally killing a patient and accelerating his death by administering analgesic drugs, even though the hastening of death is merely foreseen. He regards drawing any moral distinction as hypocritical and as a 'ridiculous way out of responsibility'. (Interview, 25 July 1989) He thus elides a distinction which can be crucial for both legal and moral purposes. For example, in English law, the doctor who intentionally kills his patient to alleviate pain commits the offence of murder; by contrast, if the doctor intends solely to alleviate pain and the acceleration of death is an undesired side-effect, even though it is foreseen as certain, he does not. See Robert Goff, 'The Mental Element in the Crime of Murder' (1988) 104 *LOR* 30, 44–6. For a discussion of the ethical distinction which can exist see *The Principle of Respect for Human Life* (Linacre Centre Paper 1) London: The Linacre Centre, 1978 and *Is there a morally significant difference between killing and letting die*? (Linacre Centre Paper 2) London: The Linacre Centre, 1978. See generally John Finnis, 'Intention and side-effects' in R G Frey and Christopher W Morris (eds), *Liability: New Essays in Legal Philosophy* Cambridge: Cambridge University Press 1991, 32.
114 *Op. cit.* n4, *supra*, 35.

115 *NJ* (1985) No 106 451 at 452.

116 *Op. cit.* n13, *supra*, 449.

117 Marian H N Driesse *et al.*, 'Euthanasia and the Law in the Netherlands' (1988) 3 *Issues in Law & Medicine* 385, 386–7.

118 *Ibid*, 387.

119 *NJ* (1987) No 607 at 2131. In his annotation of the *Alkmaar* case, Professor van Veen comments: "there might be situations in which also the non-physician might appeal successfully to necessity. In his case, an appeal to psychological constraint [*psychische dwang*] would much rather apply than an appeal to emergency in the sense of 'conflict of duties'." *NJ* (1985) No 106 451 at 467.

120 *Op. cit.* n7, *supra*, 10.

121 See e.g. Henriette D C Roscam Abbing, 'Dying with Dignity, and Euthanasia: A View from the Netherlands' (1988) 4 *Journal of Palliative Care* 70.

122 *Op. cit.* n7, *supra*, 1.

123 *Ibid*, 7.

124 See text at n65, *supra*. An example of this is to be found in a letter to the editors of the *Hastings Center Report* in reply to the article by Fenigsen. *Op. cit.* n98, *supra*. Signed by many of the leading defenders of the Dutch approach to euthanasia it cites Leenen's definition and then states that 'euthanasia' is, therefore, necessarily voluntary, and adds that the killing of incompetent patients is not a part of the euthanasia problem. 'Letter', *ibid*.

125 Interview, 11 July 1989.

126 *Ibid*.

127 'Final Report of the Netherlands State Commission on Euthanasia: An English Summary', (1987) 1 *Bioethics* 163, 168.

128 Vision, 3.

129 *Discussienota Inzake levensbeeindigend handelen bij wilsonbekwame patienten, deel 1: zwaar-defecte pasgeborenen (Discussion paper on the termination of life of severely handicapped new-born infants)* (1988), cited by Sluyters, *op. cit.* n4, *supra*, 35.

130 Interview, Gunning, 2 August 1989.

131 Personal communication from Gunning, 27 April 1991, about the second report (entitled 'Treatment of Patients in Prolonged Coma') of the KNMG's Committee on the Acceptability of Life-ending Treatment.

132 Interview, 27 July 1989. Similarly, H M Dupuis, Professor of Medical Ethics at the University of Leiden and ex-President of the DVES, has said that she accepts that in some cases in which the diagnosis was clear, the life of an irreversibly comatose patient ought to be terminated as when stopping treatment merely increased the patient's suffering and there was a consensus that the patient's life was senseless. (Interview, 28 July 1989. See also 'The Right to a Gentle Death' in *op. cit.* n26, *supra*, 53, 55–6). Again, Tromp-Meesters, asked whether the requirement of a request did not deprive those too young or too old to make a request of a right to be relieved of suffering replied: 'Yes, I think so, and that could never be, in my view, the decision of one doctor; that should be a team of two of three people'. She added that her Society had not ruled out non-voluntary euthanasia and was still considering the matter. (Interview, 11 July 1989).

133 C van der Meer, 'Euthanasia: A Definition and Ethical Conditions' (1988) 4 *Journal of Palliative Care* 103, 104.

134 *Op. cit.* n74, *supra*, 468–9.

135 *Ibid*, 451–67.
136 *Ibid*, 467.
137 See text at nn122–3.
138 *Op. cit.* n10, *supra*, 162.
139 *Op. cit.* n7, *supra*, 7–8.
140 See text at n123.
141 Interview, Martens, 11 July 1989.
142 'Legal Aspects of Euthanasia, Assistance to Suicide and Terminating the Medical Treatment of Incompetent Patients' (Unpublished paper delivered at a Conference on Euthanasia held at the Instituut voor Gezondheidsethiek, Maastricht, 2–4 December 1990) 6.
143 *Ibid*, 11.
144 Free Press, 1991. My review of this book appears in 22/2 (1992) *Hastings Center Report*.
145 *Ibid*, xiv.
146 *Ibid*. 121.
147 *Ibid*, 122.
148 *Ibid*, 124–5.
149 *Ibid*, 133.

7

Is there a policy for the elderly needing long-term care?

GRAHAM MULLEY

It is clear where most of us would like to live when we are old. We would naturally wish to stay in our own homes and would only consider going into residential, nursing home or long-stay hospital accommodation as a last resort. It is difficult to provide a truly satisfying quality of care in continuing-care facilities and many old people who are in these places would prefer not to be there.

Long-term institutional care should be considered only after all other options have been thoroughly explored (Greengross 1987). It should be a carefully planned positive choice. Continuing care in institutions for the elderly should be available for those who actively want it and really need it. If this form of placement is appropriate, it should be provided in a supportive, homely environment where the individual's autonomy and privacy can be respected and where people can enjoy a good quality of life and high standards of care.

Ensuring that long-stay care is indicated and that the care provided is of the highest order requires careful strategic planning. Strategy originally meant the skill of a general: it was the art of conducting a military campaign by preparing and utilising forces so that the initiative would be secured and the war won. In the non-military world of planning care for the elderly, we consider strategic planning to involve a philosophy, principles and a set of values.

Strategic planning requires a map, which shows us where we want to be, and a route, indicating the ways in which we can reach our destination. It demands a statement of desired outcomes and tools to measure whether these outcomes have been achieved.

This survey of the development of long-term care of the elderly in the United Kingdom will show that politicians and health professionals have not set out long-term intentions or devised plans of action for the most

101

disadvantaged members of our ageing population. The needs of the chronically ill who depend on others have not been considered as carefully as the needs of the acutely ill or those requiring rehabilitation. Political ideology, inadequate medical training and negative attitudes have resulted in a fragmented pattern of inappropriate care. Many old people go into institutions who do not need this type of support and much state and private money is spent on providing long-stay accommodation in which the quality of care is often sub-optimal. Let us see how this unhappy situation has arisen.

Warehouses for the aged

In the sixteenth century, those impoverished old people who required care were often placed in the workhouse and those deemed mentally ill were put into asylums. In these places, all aspects of life were regimented. Everyone in these harsh institutions was obliged to lead a highly structured existence. Routines were strict and officials imposed formal rules (Goffman 1961).

In the eighteenth and nineteenth centuries, two distinct types of hospital came into being. The voluntary hospitals concentrated on acute and 'interesting' cases. They developed specialist services, gained kudos and had no difficulty in attracting well-educated nurses who wished to be trained to high standards of professionalism. By contrast, the poor law hospitals provided care for those incapacitated by chronic disease, who were excluded from or who had been discharged from the voluntary hospitals. Recruitment was difficult, and nursing in these less favoured hospitals was considered to be a craft rather than a profession (Adams 1964). The medical profession generally showed little interest in the occupants of the wards of these hospitals, assuming that nothing could be done for these patients. The management of these 'incurables' tended to be uninvolved and perfunctory. Standards of care were often low as was staff morale. Many of these wards for the chronic sick were to become the seedbeds from which geriatric medicine was to grow and flourish.

A new medical speciality

Poor Law Hospitals were medical backwaters, often situated some distance from the voluntary hospitals. They were poorly designed, inadequately equipped and overcrowded. The patients were considered to be 'social' or 'chronic' cases rather than 'medical' patients.

During the Second World War, a small group of doctors began to question the received wisdom about these elderly invalids who were tended on understaffed long-stay wards. Led by Marjorie Warren in London, these pioneering geriatricians discovered that some of the patients who had been consigned to permanent hospital care had potentially treatable medical conditions. Unhappily, these patients had never been fully assessed. Enforced immobility had resulted in contractures and pressure sores which compounded their misery and invalidity. By applying basic principles of medicine, nursing and rehabilitation, creating a positive ambience and a more pleasant physical environment, it was found that many of these people improved to such an extent that they no longer required hospital care (Williamson 1979).

Having recognised that many long-stay patients suffered from preventable diseases or disorders that could have been minimised by early intervention, the physicians in the new speciality of geriatric medicine sought to reduce the development of unnecessary disability and dependence by early assessment and treatment. By working as part of an inter-disciplinary team, recognising and orchestrating the skills of nurses, therapists, social workers and others, and changing traditional nihilistic and ageist attitudes held by health professionals, geriatricians have made enormous improvements in the health care of the elderly.

By home assessment, early referrals, careful discharge planning and provision of community support, the management of ill old people has been revolutionised. There are now undergraduate and postgraduate training programmes and a Royal College of Physicians Diploma in Geriatric Medicine. Much excellent research work is focussed on old age.

Medicine for the elderly now takes place in district general hospitals as well as teaching hospitals, where the main emphasis of clinical work is on prevention, acute care and rehabilitation. The length of hospital stay for sick old people has been greatly reduced and most are successfully treated and are able to return home. Geriatric medicine has become a major branch of medicine. There has probably never been a better time to be old and ill.

But what of those who do not make a good recovery and are not restored to independence? Most are still able to go home, where they are usually supported by families and other carers, including members of the health and social services. Some will require alternative forms of care. When the National Health Service began in 1948, it was believed that old people who required long-term care could be neatly categorised: the chronic sick, who would be looked after by the health service, and the frail elderly, who would be the responsibility of the local authority. The chronic sick were managed in long-stay wards, the frail elderly in social service residential homes (also known as aged person's homes, rest homes, eventide homes, or part III accommodation). Whilst the treatment of old people with acute medical problems and the rehabilitation of the disabled elderly took place on active wards, with a positive atmosphere, those who required continuing hospital care fared less well.

Long-stay hospital wards

Most long-stay elderly patients who live in hospital do so in old-fashioned wards, some of which were former isolation wards or sanatoria. They are usually of a 'Nightingale' design – open wards, in which all the beds can be easily seen by the nurses. Though observation of patients is maximised, this style of care deprives people of a normal domestic pattern of living. There is little or no personal space where they can entertain friends or be alone. The decor is often clinical and stark, the environment unnecessarily institutional (Horrocks 1986). There may be no carpets or curtains, few flowers, photographs or mementoes. Windows may be too high: wheelchair users' view of the outside world may be limited to a glimpse of the sky. Although good quality care can be provided on these wards, standards are sometimes low. The staff may concentrate on the patients' physical needs, with less emphasis on social, emotional and spiritual aspects of care.

Patients may be denied autonomy: they may have no choice of food, clothing, activities, bedtimes. These wards often have few trained nurses who may receive little medical support.

Given this unhappy combination of inadequate, outmoded buildings, inappropriately designed and poorly furnished; a paucity of committed, enthusiastic and well-trained staff and a dearth of medical interest, it is hardly surprising that the quality of care and the quality of life on these wards may be far from satisfactory. This is exemplified by a number of scandals which have sporadically focussed attention on the plight of long-stay hospital patients.

The Health Advisory Service (Age Concern England 1990) has reported that the quality of care in some units is devastatingly low. In some, the thoughtless use of physical restraints is widespread. Urinary incontinence is untreated or inadequately managed; catheterisation rates are unacceptably high. The daily routine may be geared more to the convenience of the staff than to the needs of the patients. Because of poor working conditions and low standards, staff recruitment is difficult. Sickness absence is high, often as a result of lifting injuries. Some wards contain an inappropriate combination of patients: younger disabled people and those with rheumatological, orthopaedic and dermatological problems may be grouped with long-stay geriatric patients.

Private nursing homes

In recent years, there has been a dramatic increase in the number of private nursing homes providing care for the elderly in the United Kingdom, and a decline in the number of NHS long-stay beds. The main stimulus to this change was an alteration in the supplementary benefits system, in 1983, whereby people on low income could obtain government funding to pay for board and lodging in private nursing home or residential home care (McKie 1987). Between 1982 and 1984 there was a 36 per cent increase in the number of nursing home beds (Day & Klein 1987). The closure of large numbers of long-stay wards and the privatisation of continuing care took place without public or professional debate. It appears to have been unplanned; certainly the enormous costs to the Treasury cannot have been anticipated. Supplementary benefit payments for private care increased from £105 m in 1983 to £1300 m in 1991. The development of private facilities has not been uniform throughout the country. In Scotland, for example, there were 34 nursing home places per 100 000 total population at a time when there were 220 such places in the South East Thames health region. In some districts, the provision of private beds now exceeds those provided by the NHS: in one part of Cornwall in 1986, there were three nursing home beds to every one long-stay hospital bed. The wisdom of this development has been questioned (Coni 1987). Certainly, private nursing homes provide old people with a choice. These homes tend to be smaller and more homely than many hospital wards, and some are in the locality in which residents' families live. Many provide excellent standards of care as well as a high quality of life. There are, however, some problems:-

(1) Patients do not undergo an expert assessment before going into a private nursing home. The supplementation received is based on their financial status rather than their level of nursing need. Consequently, some people are condemned to permanent institutionalisation without it being determined whether they have remediable medical conditions or whether they could be restored to independent living by rehabilitation. In a study of 400 elderly residents in 18 private nursing homes, in Edinburgh,

28 per cent appeared to be independent in self-care (Primrose & Capewell 1986a). In Brighton, 23 per cent of nursing home residents had low levels of dependency (Bennett 1986). It appears then that at least a quarter of old people assigned to these homes do not actually require nursing care. With a full assessment and comprehensive treatment, it is likely that many could be restored to higher levels of independence and placed in alternative settings – or remain at home.

(2) Some old people who previously lived in hospital are being obliged to move to private nursing homes – even though they may have preferred to stay on long-stay wards. In some cases, the standard of care they subsequently received in private care was low; NHS monitoring of standards has not been as frequent or comprehensive as it might have been.

(3) Private nursing homes tend to take those old people who are less dependent than those who occupy long-stay wards. Although the main requirement is for facilities where the demented and physically heavily dependent patients can be cared for, nursing homes usually have a lower proportion of confused, incontinent or highly dependent patients than do hospitals (Bennett (1986); Primrose & Capewell 1986b).

(4) Once in nursing homes, old people may have difficulty obtaining services and equipment that they would have received had they been in hospital or at home. They have difficulty with the provision of walking aids and incontinence aids; they have to pay extra for physiotherapy or chiropody (Primrose & Capewell 1986c).

(5) Economic pressures on homes can militate against the provision of good standards of care. Dining rooms and lounges may be converted to bedrooms so that more people can be accommodated. In one survey, only 50 per cent of private nursing homes had day rooms, and access was often difficult because of the lack of lifts (Primrose & Capewell 1986b). Most residents have to share their bedroom with one or more people. One in four residents in Edinburgh nursing homes had neither a single bedroom nor a proper common room, a situation making it difficult for them to enjoy privacy. Economic difficulties may lead to cost-cutting: staffing levels may be inadequate, catering costs may be trimmed, equipment not purchased.

(6) Older residents of private nursing homes do not have the reassurance that this is to be their permanent home. The owners may go out of business: the home may close or change hands.

(7) Some nursing home residents do not receive basic geriatric care (MacMahon, Bhakri & Bowman 1986). The staff may feel isolated and may not be aware of advances in geriatric nursing. The need for training

and support has been emphasised (Millard 1981): if standards are to be high and the morale of staff sustained, it is essential that education and training are provided and that nurses and care assistants receive advice from therapists and specialist nurses.

We have seen how the speciality of geriatric medicine arose because patients were placed on chronic wards without a comprehensive assessment by a team of skilled and experienced health professionals. It is regrettable that the recent insidious privatisation of long-term care is depriving a significant group of old people of the opportunity to be restored to optimum levels of independence (Coni 1987).

NHS nursing homes

An alternative model of long-term care is the nursing home run by the NHS (Evans 1989). The first three such homes have been evaluated (Bond, Gregson & Atkinson 1989). They are small units, administered by nurses. Medical input is provided by general practitioners rather than consultant geriatricians. These homes provide a more satisfying environment than long-stay wards – they are more homely and offer a wider range of social and recreational activities. Despite detailed studies of the improved quality of life in these homes, there has not been a widespread provision of them. This would suggest that the government is not eager to invest in State provision of high quality long-term care, preferring to leave this to the private sector.

Residential care

In the United Kingdom, long-term care for those requiring nursing care takes place in hospitals or nursing homes. Those whose needs are not primarily for nursing and medical care, but who require supported living, may be admitted to residential homes. These may be state-run, private or organised by voluntary or religious organisations.

Long-term residential care should only be considered when full support at home has been tried and not succeeded, and when other forms of accommodation (such as sheltered housing) have been considered (Greengross 1987). Ideally, a residential home should be in the locality in which the residents previously lived – or be near their families. Admission should be carefully planned and should take place only when the old person has undergone detailed assessment by a social worker and a multi-disciplinary health team. Once in the home, the resident should enjoy as domestic a lifestyle as possible. They should be encouraged to manage their own lives so that they can maintain independence and dignity. They should be reviewed regularly to ensure that their social, psychological and medical needs are being fulfilled. The homes themselves should be subject to regular independent monitoring to ensure that standards are high. As these homes are not staffed by nurses, the care workers should not be expected to look after those who require continued nursing care.

In 1986, 2.5 per cent of the over 65s in Britain were living in local authority or private residential homes (Salvage, Jones and Vetter 1989). Although providing for a small proportion of people over retirement age, these homes consumed 50 per cent of the social service departments' expenditure (Stevenson 1989). These homes are not a cheap option: what about the levels of care in them?

(1) Pre-admission assessments

In a survey of one-fifth of old people admitted to residential homes in Manchester, one in three were felt by medical assessors to require alternative forms of care (Brocklehurst *et al.* 1978). In a subsequent survey in Edinburgh, seven per cent of 688 subjects being assessed for residential care were either too fit or unfit for residential care (Rafferty, Smith & Williamson 1987). In some places there is now routine multi-disciplinary screening of all applicants for residential care. This should be standard practice.

(2) Quality of care

Those residents who are mobile, articulate and independent may enjoy a satisfactory quality of life in residential care. Those who are disabled, frail or confused may be less fortunate. Although residential homes were built and staffed to provide care for retired people needing social support, many of them now house high proportions of dependent very old people. In one survey, 41 per cent of residents were incontinent of urine, 25 per cent incontinent of faeces and 4 per cent were totally dependent for their basic daily needs (Bennett 1986). In another study, 11 per cent of residents were chairfast or bedfast, 10 per cent required help with walking and 10 per cent were doubly incontinent (McLaughlan & Wilkin 1982).

These problems of incontinence, immobility and dependence often reflect underlying physical or psychiatric illness. In a survey of 331 residents of residential homes in Liverpool (Gosney, Tallis & Edmond 1990/91), it was found that over 90 per cent had serious conditions, the commonest being cardiovascular, psychiatric and rheumatological disorders. Many of these people ought to receive regular medical reviews: their condition may gradually deteriorate, and the side-effects of medication ought to be monitored. Nearly one in ten receive inappropriate medication and are therefore at risk of adverse drug reactions. Yet residents of local authority homes are not usually monitored by general practitioners and regular assessments by district nurses, geriatric health visitors or community psychiatric nurses are rare.

Many residents are confused and some have behavioural problems. Yet the levels and training of staff mean that many of these residents will not receive optimum care. Perhaps by default, we have created what have become in effect local authority nursing homes staffed by people who usually have no medical or nursing training and which have few opportunities for detailed review by a multi-disciplinary team or for rehabilitation.

(3) Quality of life

The homes run by Social Service departments have separate dining rooms and most provide day rooms and single bedrooms (Bennett 1986). In these homes, the residents can feel secure and comfortable and have the freedom to be private when they choose. The staff are often very committed, caring people who are busy doing exhausting, unpopular work for low rates of pay. Low staffing levels mean that residents cannot always attain the quality of life that is desirable. They should be able to get up when they want, but there may not be enough staff to get frail residents up and dressed in time for breakfast. Encouraging people to do things independently often takes more time than assisting them. Staff are so busy feeding, dressing, bathing and toiletting people that they may not have enough time to listen, talk or provide mental stimulation (Sinclair 1988). Many residents are lonely and bored. It is thought to be a good thing to place chairs in groups in a day room to facilitate socialisation; but a clear majority of those who expressed a preference like to have their chairs lined up against the wall (Willcocks *et al.* 1982). People should have the freedom not to be sociable, should they so wish.

The burden of caring for elderly residents can be too much, especially if the staff are untrained and become intolerant and impatient under stress. Scandals such as that at Nye Bevan Lodge in Southwark, where some

residential home staff practised 'extortion, torture and blackmail' under-
line the need for better training, higher staffing levels and regular
independent monitoring of these homes (McKie 1987).

In general, local authority residential homes are favoured by the
Labour party and private nursing homes by the Conservatives. The left
wing view is that public provision is good, but private care is not, being
operated by people who are motivated largely by greed. There have
certainly been scandals in private residential homes, just as there have
been malpractices in local authority homes. A recent editorial in *The
Independent* (1991) stated that conditions in some private homes were
shamefully bad; particular concern was voiced about the disgraceful and
humiliating lack of privacy. In some homes, elderly residents were obliged
to use commodes, get undressed and bathe in front of strangers.

These are the exception; in most cases, private rest homes provide a
homely, clean and warm environment where there is much activity and
close contact between staff and residents (Andrews 1984; Snape 1984). In
the few homes providing poor care, there was an odour of stale urine;
residents were restrained in 'geriatric' chairs; Christmas decorations were
still hanging in June.

Other problems have been identified in private residential homes:-

Forty per cent of residents are admitted directly from their own homes,
without being properly assessed (Snape 1984).
Many smaller homes are single sex (usually taking ladies only) (Lowrey
& Briggs 1988).
The district nurse services are reluctant to provide gadgets and equip-
ment that residents would have received had they been in their own
homes – examples being toilet aids, bath aids, commodes, special
mattresses (Andrews 1984).
Many private homes have few or no single rooms or dayrooms.
Though the residents may be confused or incontinent, the staff may not
receive basic training which would enable them to provide better care
(Andrews 1984).
Residents whose medical problems would be better managed in nursing
homes or hospital sometimes stay in the rest home.
Inspections – which would usually be welcomed by home owners – are
rare and not very rigorous.

Of particular concern are large amounts of money that have been
channelled into residential care for people with a generally low level of
dependency. This money would have been far better spent on detailed

pre-admission assessments and increased domiciliary support. As a result of this governmental blunder, large numbers of old people have been unnecessarily institutionalised and too little financial provision has been made available for community support.

Conclusions

The lay person's view of a doctor who specialises in the care of old people who suffer from physical or psychological problems is of someone providing custodial care of the elderly. Yet from the inception of the speciality of geriatric medicine, doctors have been more concerned with acute medicine and rehabilitation than providing high quality care for those who require long-term support. The small number of pages in geriatric textbooks devoted to the consideration of long-term care and the relatively few research publications devoted to the improvement of the lot of these patients, is testimony to the relative lack of interest shown by doctors in very disabled old people who have chronic illness. Clearly, the doctor's role in long-term care is far less important than that of the nurse or care assistant and it is important not to medicalise long-term care when a domestic rather than a clinical ambience is more appropriate. Nonetheless, the medical profession has a number of important roles here, not least in helping to shape strategic planning.

In Britain, we have a 400-year tradition of placing our poorest, most dependent and oldest people into lack-lustre settings where they have often received low quality care. Neither health professionals nor politicians have set out long term intentions or devised a plan of action for the provision of appropriate, imaginative and humane care of the most disadvantaged members of our ageing population. Perhaps we are now beginning to learn from our past mistakes and develop a clearer idea of what needs to be done. Long-term geriatric care has not been a source of national pride. It is now time to rectify this.

References

Adams, G. F. (1964). 'Nursled' survival. *Lancet*, **2**, 303–4.

Age Concern England (1990). Left behind? Continuing care for the elderly people in NHS hospitals. *A review of Health Advisory Service reports.* London: Age Concern England.

Andrews, K. (1984). Private rest homes in the care of the elderly. *British Medical Journal*, **288**, 1518–20.

Bennett, J. (1986). Private nursing homes: contribution to long stay care of the elderly in the Brighton Health District. *British Medical Journal*, **293**, 867–70.

Bond, J., Gregson, B. A. & Atkinson, A. (1989). Measurement of outcomes within a multicentred randomised controlled trial in the evaluation of the experimental NHS nursing homes. *Age and Ageing*, **18**, 292–302.

Brocklehurst, J. C., Carty, M. H., Leeming, J. T. & Robinson, J. M. (1978). Medical screening of old people accepted for residential care. *Lancet*, **2**, 141–3.

Coni, N. K. (1987). Private homes for elderly patients. *Lancet*, **2**, 102.

Day, P. & Klein, R. (1987). Quality of institutional care and the elderly: policy issues and options. *British Medical Journal*, **294**, 384–7.

Evans, J. G. (1989). National Health Service Nursing Homes. *Age and Ageing*, **18**, 289–91.

Goffman, E. (1961). *Asylum: essays on the social situation of mental patients and other inmates*. New York: Anchor.

Gosney, M., Tallis, R. & Edmond, E. (1990/91). The burden of chronic illness in local authority residential homes for the elderly. *Health Trends*, **4**, 153–7.

Greengross, S. (1987). Political action and advocacy. *Danish Medical Bulletin*. Gerontology Special Supplement Series No 5. pp. 68–73.

Horrocks, P. (1986). The components of a comprehensive district health service for elderly people – a personal view. *Age and Ageing*, **15**, 321–42.

The Independent (1991). Shameful care for the elderly. 31 January p. 22.

Lowrey, S. & Briggs, R. (1988). Boom in private rest homes in Southampton: impact on the elderly in residential care. *British Medical Journal*, **296**, 541–3.

McKie, D. (1987). Much disquiet again about residential homes for the elderly. *Lancet*, **2**, 287–8.

McLauchlan, S. & Wilkin, D. (1982). Levels of provision and of dependency in residential homes for the elderly: implications for planning. *Health Trends*, **14**, 63–5.

MacMahon, D. G., Bhakri, H. L. & Bowman, C. E. (1986). Nursing dependency in registered nursing homes and long term geriatric wards. *British Medical Journal*, **293**, 265–6.

Millard, P. H. (1981). Last scene of all. *British Medical Journal*, **283**, 1559–60.

Primrose, W. R. & Capewell, A. E. (1986, a). A survey of registered nursing homes within the city of Edinburgh. *Journal of the Royal College of General Practitioners*, **36**, 125–8.

Primrose, W. R. & Capewell, A. E. (1986, b). Private nursing homes: contribution to long stay care. *British Medical Journal*, **293**, 1306–7.

Primrose, W. R. & Capewell, A. E. (1986, c). Private nursing homes and the old. *Lancet*, **1**, 99.

Rafferty, J., Smith, R. G. & Williamson, J. (1987). Medical assessment of elderly patients prior to a move to residential care: a review of seven years' experience in Edinburgh. *Age and Ageing*, **16**, 10–12.

Salvage, A. V., Jones, D. A. & Vetter, N. J. (1989). Opinions of people aged over 75 years on private and local authority residential care. *Age and Ageing*, **18**, 380–6.

Sinclair, I. (editor) (1988). *Residential Care: The Research Reviewed*. Literature surveys commissioned by the Independent Review of Residential Care. London: HMSO.

Snape, J. (1984). Private rest homes. *British Medical Journal*, **289**, 381–2.

Stevenson, O. (1989). *Age and vulnerability. A guide to better care*. London: Edward Arnold.

Willcocks, D., Ring, J., Kellaher, L. and Peace, S. (1982). The Residential Life of Old People. A study of 100 Local Authority Homes. Vol II: Appendices. Polytechnic of North London: Survey Research Unit.

Williamson, J. (1979). Notes on the historical development of geriatric medicine as a medical speciality. *Age and Ageing*, **8**, 144–8.

8

Is it possible to provide good quality long-term care without unfair discrimination?

ROBERT STOUT

This paper describes some areas of difficulty which may occur in providing high quality long-stay care to everybody who needs it. Whether this is discrimination or not depends how broad a definition is given to this term.

Provision of resources

In order to provide high quality long-term care the first need is to have the proper facilities. This is not a matter which is under the control of doctors and is very much dependent on financial resources being made available by health authorities and boards and ultimately by the Government. A striking feature of health care is that very expensive high technology equipment is often readily available, and public appeals are sometimes used to provide this, but the technology of long-term care of elderly people, namely well designed and well staffed wards, is much less easy to obtain and does not excite the generosity of the public. When the distribution of wards within hospitals is decided, it is often the oldest and least attractive parts of the hospital that are allocated to those who are going to be in hospital longest, indeed, for whom hospital is going to be their home. The medical profession itself, and particularly that part of it which works in hospital, has a major responsibility for these attitudes. General practitioners appear to be much more alert to the needs of dependent elderly people than doctors working in the acute hospital specialties, and it is these who often have a major influence on the distribution of resources within hospitals.

It is also true that the workload per doctor, per nurse or per therapist is often greater in geriatric units than in other hospital departments, suggesting perhaps that other specialities are overstaffed rather than that care of the elderly is understaffed. Some re-distribution of resources would be appropriate. Unfortunately, re-distribution of resources now more often means reductions in resources rather than the distribution of new resources and here again geriatric long-stay units are particularly vulnerable.

In the last decade an additional resource for dependent elderly people has become widely available in the form of private nursing homes. A controlled transfer of the care of at least some elderly people from the statutory to the private sector is not objectionable, provided there has been full public debate and agreement on this. Not only has there not been debate and agreement, the new provisions for community care, which would make such a transfer easier and the new arrangements more acceptable, have been postponed until 1993 for reasons which have nothing to do with the health care of dependent elderly people.

Choice

In recent Government documents, not only on Health but also on other subjects such as Education, emphasis is placed on consumer choice. This may have the unfortunate effect of raising unrealistic expectations, as absolute choice, particularly when resources are limited, is impossible. In the care of dependent elderly people choice is a particularly difficult concept when emphasis is also placed on assessment of need and appropriate use of resources. A simple example, familiar to all doctors responsible for managing geriatric beds, is of the elderly patient previously living in poor circumstances and dependent on a close relative for help, who is admitted to hospital as an emergency, recovers and refuses to be discharged. Hospital care is no longer needed and a bed which should be used by somebody else in greater need continues to be occupied. The new community care initiative does not seem to cover this circumstance. There is an ethical, as well as to some extent legal, dilemma in dealing with this situation. When availability of alternatives to long-stay geriatric beds was less, such patients would probably have remained in hospital. Now, however, managers of scarce resources could not justify such a patient remaining in hospital. So what does choice mean? And how can the proper use of resources be enforced?

While choice has always been limited in National Health Service continuing care wards, it is one of the often-stated advantages of the private sector, so long as the patient or his family can find the money to pay the charges. There is no requirement to demonstrate need for the type of care provided. This will change under the new arrangements for community care, at least for those whose stay is supported by statutory funds. When funds are transferred from Social Security to Local Authorities, assessment of need will be instituted. Choice will be further restricted, although perhaps justifiably.

Ability to pay

In the National Health Service long-stay care is provided without consideration of the patient's ability to pay. The State Pension is reduced after a period of time in hospital and thus pensioners are the only people who have to pay for their care in hospital in the National Health Service. Other financial resources are not considered. Although reduction in the state pension may seem reasonable when care, food and warmth are provided by a state funded service, loss of one pension to an elderly couple may cause financial hardship. For statutory residential care there has always been a requirement for the resident to pay what he can afford and means testing takes place, taking into account all financial assets. This is sometimes a disincentive to elderly people or their relatives for a move from hospital to statutory residential care. Nevertheless, if the elderly person has no significant financial resources, neither she nor her relatives are required to find money to supplement the costs.

The situation has become more complicated with the widespread use of private nursing and residential care. Here the charges are set by the proprietors. Currently, Social Security funds are available to provide fixed amounts depending on the patient's assets and degree of dependency. However, charges depend on market forces. If the supply of nursing home places is greater than the supply of available clients, charges are held down. If there is a demand for places, charges are high. Sometimes newly opened nursing homes admit the first few patients at Social Security levels but rapidly increase the charges for later admissions, or indeed seek to increase the charges for their early patients at a later date.

There are a number of concerns about this approach. For example, the question as to whether the patient remains in hospital accommodation or moves to a private nursing home is very much related to the ability and willingness of the patient and often the family to pay what can be substantial amounts of money. In general, those who have no means and who can be supported by Social Security funds are not too troubled and a home which accepts them at Social Security level can usually be found. Presumably those who have substantial means are also largely untroubled. For those with modest means, which are often tied up in a house or, even more significantly, in rural areas, in a farm which is expected to be passed on through the generations of the family, this may be a substantial disincentive to using the private sector. This is an area which has not received widespread public debate. Indeed, the whole subject of whether old people can expect to hand down assets to their family or must use them to support themselves should be publicly debated. This is also a concern in other countries. Speaking of long-term care, the United States Secretary of Health and Human Services has said: 'We must decide how much we should ask people to contribute to the cost of their care, particularly people whose wealth would otherwise permit them to pay for most of their care out of pocket. We must further address an important philosophical issue that all of us in society must deal with   the extent to which public long-term care policy should support the understandable and natural desire of older people to pass on some of their wealth to their children'.[1] A second concern is whether those homes which, for market or other reasons, hold their costs down will be able to maintain adequate standards. A third concern is that homes which may have different rates for different clients may discriminate between the clients. Residents who pay for themselves and those supported by Social Security may be segregated and the former may have single rooms while the latter have to share accommodation. Most people would find this type of discrimination unacceptable and quite contrary to what they are used to in the hospital sector, although perhaps something like this will be coming into the market-style National Health Service. It is interesting to consider why this type of discrimination is considered repugnant when it is accepted that people live in different standards of houses, drive different types of cars and take different types of holidays, all according to what they can afford.

If long-term care for the most dependent elderly people moves from a system where it is largely supplied by the National Health Service to one where it is largely or even totally supplied by the private sector, these issues are going to become more important. It is, as mentioned before, a matter of serious concern that the moves that are occurring in this direction are being carried out without public debate and without apparently any firm policy direction. Changes will occur when the new policies for community care are introduced but while some of the practical arrangements may change, the issues that have been outlined will remain.

Mental state and dependency

It is a normal human response to find caring for some people more enjoyable and more worthwhile than caring for others. This is not simply a measure of the amount of work that patients require but is probably related more to patient's personalities, their expressions of gratitude, their willingness to try to help themselves, and their tolerance of suffering. It is inevitable that nurses and doctors will be more drawn to some patients than to others for these reasons. Patient's relatives also may have an influence and relatives who are persistently critical and complaining will antagonise staff and may cause negative attitudes towards patients. While patients whose mental capacity is impaired have particular management problems, mental impairment does not necessarily result in a difficult personality or correlate with how well patients are liked. In the National Health Service patients are admitted according to their need and geriatric units find themselves dealing with the most dependent as well as the most difficult patients. In order to cope with these difficult patients, staff must be present in adequate numbers and must be well motivated. However, until now patients who require intensive nursing or who have difficult personalities have been present in relatively small numbers among other patients whose nursing requirements are less or who are more agreeable. One of the potential problems of the increasing use of the private sector is that the mix of patients in hospital continuing care wards will change. Nursing homes are under no obligation to take anybody, apart from their need to balance income with expenditure, and when the demand exceeds the number of places they will usually be selective in taking those whose needs are less and who are easier to manage. If this continues it may happen that National Health Service continuing care wards will have a high concentration of the most difficult patients and patients who are easy to manage will be in the private sector. This will have two deleterious effects. First the quality of life for patients in continuing care wards will diminish. Second recruitment and retention of high quality staff will become more difficult. It is of course wrong to use patients as pawns in order to improve the conditions for staff and nobody is advocating this. Nevertheless, this problem may have to be faced and appropriate incentives for staff in very high dependency geriatric units will have to be considered.

Need

Ideally high quality long-term care should be provided on the basis of need. Need is difficult to define and almost impossible to measure, given the variability between individuals. Need involves both the physical and mental condition of the patient, which he may or may not give expression to, and which potential carers may or may not have the ability and desire to meet. It is difficult to relate services to need. Some people with the highest degrees of dependency receive the highest quality care at home from totally untrained carers. One of the aims of the speciality of geriatric medicine is that nobody is admitted to long-term care unless every effort at treatment and rehabilitation has been exhausted and all other possible settings have been explored. Care in the community, now promulgated by the Government, has always been the philosophy of geriatric medicine. Need as judged by specialists in geriatric medicine is the criterion which is applied to the allocation of National Health Service long-term care facilities. Despite this, a recent survey of elderly patients in geriatric long-stay beds in South Belfast revealed every degree of dependency from one independent patient to a majority who were highly dependent.[2] Thus, measures of dependency do not identify all characteristics of need, especially personality factors. The wilfully dependent are another problem.

In the private sector need for care is not currently a criterion for allocation of resources to individuals. Availability of a place and of financial resources to pay for it are all that are required. A further survey in South Belfast showed that dependency levels of nursing home residents were similar to those of residents in statutory residential care but considerably lower than patients in geriatric continuing care wards.[3] It seems, therefore, that there are people in nursing homes who do not need nursing care and that places in nursing homes, in many cases supported by public funds, may be used inappropriately. If resources are limited, this could deprive those in need of places in nursing homes. When the new policies for community care are implemented, assessment of need will be required before public funds are used to support nursing home care. Ideally, the assessment should include an examination by a specialist in geriatric medicine so that disease and disability are recognised and treatment and rehabilitation used appropriately with perhaps removal of the need for nursing care.

Long-stay care will also be inappropriate if it has to be supplied because of inadequate treatment or rehabilitation. A recent study in the USA showed that the introduction of a prospective payment system which limits the funds available for hospital treatment of any condition (diagnosis related groups (DRG)) resulted in elderly patients with hip fractures having shorter lengths of stay in hospital, less physiotherapy, being able to walk less well on discharge from hospital, and having more admissions and more prolonged stays in nursing homes than occurred with previous more flexible systems of payment.[4] 'Efficiency' of hospital care may lead to discrimination against the patient.

Limitations of treatment

The question of how actively treatment should be applied to patients whose dependency level is such that they require continuing care in hospital can be difficult to answer. The most dramatic example of this is cardiopulmonary resuscitation. As with so many of these apparent ethical dilemmas, a review of the established facts limits the choices more than many people realise. In the literature, successful cardiopulmonary resuscitation is usually defined as the patient leaving hospital alive. If this definition is used, successful cardiopulmonary resuscitation is impossible in continuing care patients as well as in patients who are residents of nursing homes and perhaps of residential homes as well. The success rate of cardiopulmonary resuscitation in even the best centres is low, somewhere around 10% and the adverse prognostic factors are now well established. They include the co-existence of other serious diseases, including pneumonia and renal failure, a disabled state and previous housebound existence. Any of these reduce the chances of success considerably and a combination reduces the success rate to almost nil. These of course are all likely to feature prominently in patients in continuing care wards. The argument is sometimes used that cardiopulmonary resuscitation might as well be tried as 'there is nothing to lose'. What is lost in an unsuccessful resuscitation attempt is dignity in dying, as well as the peace of mind of other patients, relatives and staff. The choices here are fairly clear and the decisions almost make themselves. This is not discrimination based on age but a realistic appraisal of both the means and ends of a particular type of treatment.

Less easy are decisions on other types of supportive therapy such as antibiotics, intravenous or naso-gastric fluids or the use of modern but expensive and largely unproven methods for preventing or treating pressure sores. Nobody would deny patients who have simple reversible illnesses the treatment they need even if they are receiving continuing care in hospital, nor would symptomatic relief be questioned. However, the use of supportive treatment in patients who have progressive and irremediable conditions, with the possibility of recovery having been ruled out, is much less easy to justify. In the patient with an acute stroke whose unconsciousness persists beyond the early stages, supportive treatment may merely prolong a vegetative state, perhaps without suffering for the patient, although this is uncertain, but certainly increasing the suffering for the relatives. If it is accepted that such supportive therapy is only justifiable as a temporary measure to allow the patient to survive a transient and treatable episode so that recovery can then occur, the decisions are less difficult. It was never intended that these measures should be used as permanent life support for patients with irremediable conditions.

Another example of high-cost high technology is haemodialysis. Is it justifiable to maintain patients with chronic renal failure on haemodialysis so that they can continue to exist in a continuing care ward? This question is likely to arise more often now that dialysis is becoming available for older patients. Because of this, collaborative geriatric/ nephrology services should be introduced to consider the older patients who are now coming to the attention of nephrologists.

Paramount in all this should be the patient's wishes but it may be impossible to ascertain the wishes of patients receiving long-term care who often have widespread brain damage either from degenerative or vascular disease, and they have not usually expressed their views in advance. Families will often say that they know that their relatives would not wish to live in a severely disabled state and this information should be taken seriously.

None of these considerations involves discrimination on the basis of age. They are examples of considering the aims of treatment in the context of the patient's life and prognosis. Indeed, the thoughtless use of medical technology, irrespective of the benefits, is itself discriminatory. One of the benefits of the speciality of geriatric medicine should be the avoidance of the elderly patient being over-investigated, under-diagnosed and over-treated as may occur in other parts of the health service. Wider public debate of some of these issues would be helpful.

What is needed?

The provision of good quality care without unfair discrimination requires methods to make objective measurements of two areas – quality of care and need. Since for both of these there will always be a fairly strong subjective element, the measurements will never be exact. However, they should be much better than what is currently available. It would be appropriate for university departments of geriatric medicine to take the lead in devising such measurements. However, universities demand from their academic staff grants from the Research councils and publications in respected peer-reviewed journals and work of this type is unlikely to lead to either of these. Perhaps this is another form of discrimination.

References

1 Greenberg, D. Who pays for health care? *Lancet* (1990) **1**, 280–1.
2 Hodkinson, E., McCafferty, F. G., Scott, J. N., Stout, R. W. Disability and dependency in elderly people in residential and hospital care. *Age and Ageing* (1988) **17**, 147–54.
3 Campbell, H., Crawford, V., Stout, R. W. The impact of private residential and nursing care on statutory residential and hospital care of elderly people in South Belfast. *Age and Ageing* (1990) **19**, 318–24.
4 Fitzgerald, J. F., Moore, P. S., Dittus, R. S. The care of elderly patients with hip fracture. Changes since implementation of the prospective payment system. *New England Journal of Medicine* (1988) **319**, 1392–7.

9

The prospects for long-term care: current policy and realistic alternatives

DAVID J HUNTER

Introduction

The United Kingdom is in the midst of considerable policy turbulence in respect of health and social care provision. As a consequence, the prospects for long-term care over the next decade are unclear but potentially of considerable concern. The NHS and Community Care Act 1990 is firmly on the Statute Book and the NHS changes were introduced on 1 April 1991 as planned. But there is continuing political uncertainty and ambivalence about aspects of the reforms particularly as they impinge upon the future of community care. There is a view that the reforms do little to address the fundamental issue of who is responsible for long-term care – is it individuals, or their families, or society at large? A deep seated ambivalence about policy prevails centring not only on its content but also on its implementation.

This chapter is in three sections. The first section comprises a brief review of the position of elderly people in the UK in terms of demography and services, and puts these trends in a wider European context. The second section sets out the present state of policy in respect of long-term care for elderly people and the likely prospects over the next year or so. The final section considers some of the longer term service and funding issues which policy-makers have not really begun to address but which cannot be deferred for much longer.

The changing condition of elderly people

In recent years, the increased survival of people into advanced age has become a central concern of policy-makers. A number of countries within Europe have acknowledged the need to assess the implications for social and health resources, both human and financial, of an ageing population.

Task forces have been established to produce scenarios of likely developments and their impact on societies and economies. The Netherlands have been especially advanced in this respect. The Dutch Steering Committee on Future Health Scenarios released its report, *Ageing in the Future – Scenarios Regarding Health and Ageing, 1984–2000*, in 1985.

In its 1988 report, *Ageing Populations: The Social Policy Implications*, the Organisation for Economic Cooperation and Development (OECD) predicted that the average annual growth rate of member states' populations would decrease from 0.5% during the decade 1980–1990 to −0.3% during the decade 2040–2050. This stabilisation, and ultimately even decline, of the total population would be accompanied by substantial changes in the age structure of the population. Between 1980 and 2040, by which time the ageing of the population will have peaked, the average proportion of persons aged 65 and over will have increased from 12.2% to 21.9% of the total population while the average proportion of those aged 15 years and under will have fallen from 23.4% of the population in 1980 to 18.3% in 2050.

The most significant aspect of the growing percentage of elderly people in the population is the marked increase in those aged 85 and over. Among this group is a large number of elderly people who are severely impaired physically or mentally or both. The expansion of the elderly population has particular implications for those suffering from dementia. Estimates of the number of dementia sufferers vary considerably but the figure among those aged 85 and over has been put at 20% (Henwood 1990).

Although there is evidence of increased fitness associated with longevity, the volume of dependency among the very old will increase significantly, albeit in a generally 'fitter' older population. Demand for health and social care rises sharply with age: 1% of those aged 75–79 have severe disabilities compared with 41% of those aged 85 and over. Dependency among the over 80 year olds will increase relative to demand from smaller proportions of those aged 65–69 and 75–79 since the latter groups will be less numerous.

Need for care

Demographic trends are therefore significant and complex in their implications for long-term care. The place of informal carers (i.e. families and friends) cannot be overlooked. According to 1989 OPCS data, six million people provide informal care within the UK but the changing age structure noted earlier has a direct impact on this group. Whereas women carers in the age group 45–60 represented 63 people for every 100 persons over 65 in 1900, by 1989 the figure had fallen to 45. Over the next decade and beyond, therefore, there will be a major demand for care services coupled with a reduction in the capacity of informal carers to care. However, it is important to keep a sense of perspective and not become alarmist. Contrary to popular belief, and as has been indicated already, the majority of elderly people are neither disabled nor dependent – they live in their own homes or in those of their relatives. The greater part of health care of elderly people will be from primary health care. Most elderly people – especially the so-called 'young old' or 'well elderly' – lead full, satisfying and independent lives and will in all probability continue to do so.

The three key indicators of likely need for care among elderly people are: the fact of living alone, the inability to get in/out of bed unaided, and dementia (discussed above). Over one third of elderly people live alone including more than half of those aged 85+. Most basic functions like getting into and out of bed can be managed by all but a very small proportion of elderly people. The steep rise in inability with increasing age is evident and while the proportions are small they are not insignificant. For instance, seven per cent of all elderly people aged 85+ were unable to manage to get in/out of bed unaided compared with three per cent of those aged 80–84 and two per cent of those aged 75–79 (Henwood 1990).

A recent WHO (1989) study commented on the considerable confusion evident in discussing community and institutional long-term care. In the expert committee's view

Community care has been incorrectly proposed as a substitute for institutional care rather than as a viable part of total care, in its own right. This so-called 'alternatives mentality' has led to much unprofitable work (p. 64)

The committee argues that some people will require a more structured environment than may be available through community services. Its concern is that an emphasis on substituting community care for institutional care should not distract attention from the issue of ensuring a high quality of care in institutions. There is no clear-cut line of distinction between what care can and should be provided in the community and what is best provided in an institution. This issue goes to the nub of current policy and the changes taking place in health and social care services throughout the UK. Although successive governments have sought, through a range of policy initiatives and instruments, to achieve effectively coordinated, or seamfree, health and social care services, the reality has fallen short of policy intentions (Hunter & Wistow (eds) 1989). It is to these issues that we now turn before looking ahead to the next decade in order to assess the policy options available to policy-makers in the light of the demographic trends and the need for care outlined in this section.

Present policy

The government's stated policy on community care (long-term care in the NHS is considered in greater detail by Mulley in his chapter) as set out in the NHS and Community Care Act 1990 broadly follows the recommendations set out in the Griffiths report and subsequently modified in the 1989 White Paper, *Caring for People*. The central issue confronting those charged with implementing the reforms arises from the fact that implementation is to be phased over a three year period beginning on 1 April 1991. The overriding reason for this decision was political, aimed at maintaining control over the Community Charge bills likely to be levied by local authorities.

More recently, doubt has been cast over the government's overall strategy for community care. The decision to replace the Community Charge with a new system of local government finance coupled with the forthcoming review of the structure of local government has created renewed anxiety about the government's intentions. The Secretary of State for Health's somewhat ambiguous assertion that he could foresee no reason for the proposals not going ahead as planned has only fuelled the uncertainty. These developments, in conjunction with the delay in implementing the reforms, have created a real risk of a policy vacuum appearing in respect of community care and a continuation of the 'planning blight' which has been a persistent feature of policy in this area at least since the publication of the Griffiths review of community care in March 1988.

From Griffiths to the White Paper

In tracing the origins of the 1989 White Paper on community care, *Caring for People*, it is necessary to go back to the government's review of the whole subject carried out by its health advisor, Sir Roy Griffiths. The review was announced in late 1986 following a powerful critique of government policy carried out by the government appointed, but independent, Audit Commission. Its report, *Making a Reality of Com-*

munity Care (Audit Commission 1986), concluded that despite some £6 billion being spent on services for the priority groups, principally elderly people who consumed nearly half of this sum, progress in implementing community care was 'slow and uneven'. Five obstacles were identified to account for this state of affairs:

compartmentalised health and local authority budgets which hampered the desired shift in resources from health and social services and did not match the requirements of community care policies

the absence of bridging finance to meet the transitional costs involved in shifting from institutional to community care

the distorting effects of the public funding of private residential care which is currently (i.e. March 1991) running at around £1300 million and growing; perversely, this serves as an incentive for residential and nursing home care rather than the stated preference for domiciliary care

delays, difficulties and boundary problems caused by a fragmented organisational structure

the absence of staffing and training arrangements to ensure an appropriate supply of trained community based staff, and to ease the transfer of staff into the community.

Few of these problems are new. Many of them have existed for over 20 years. The government's response to the Audit Commission's critique was to invite Sir Roy Griffiths to review the use of public funds in supporting community care, and to advise 'on the options for action that would improve the use of these funds as a contribution to more effective care'. He reported in March 1988 (Griffiths 1988).

The Griffiths agenda is summarised in Table 1. Only the key issues are mentioned here. For a fuller discussion see Hunter & Judge (1988). In essence, Griffiths endorsed the Audit Commission's diagnosis of the problems. His starting point is the needs of individuals. They should: receive the right services in good time; have a greater say in what is done to help them and a wider choice; and be helped to stay in their own homes for as long as possible. To secure these policy ends, Griffiths proposed a realignment of responsibilities between health and local authorities, with local authority social services departments (SSDs) effectively becoming the lend agency for managing, funding, planning and regulating services locally.

Griffiths is careful to distinguish between these essentially case management functions and the actual provision of services which, in his view,

Table 1. *The Griffiths agenda*

A clearer strategic role for central government including a Minister for Community Care

A more facilitative and enabling role for social services departments as lead agencies

The continuing need for collaboration at local level between different agencies including the development of care management

New methods of financing community care including a specific community care grant

A single gateway to publicly-financed residential care

Greater encouragement for experiments to promote new forms of more pluralist provision

Restricting housing involvement to a 'bricks and mortar' role

Encouraging joint or shared training between different professions

Exploring the introduction of community carers to carry out basic care tasks

Establishing a better balance between policy aspirations and the availability of resources

Facilitating more consumer choice

Clarifying the respective responsibilities of health and social care

---

Source: Hunter & Judge (1988)

should not necessarily be the sole responsibility of monopoly public bodies. SSDs should be encouraged to move to an enabling role in order to stimulate a variety of new forms of service provision which might be provided by a variety of independent agencies. Although intent upon clarifying that which is unambiguously health and that which falls into the category of social care, Griffiths asserts that there will continue to be a need for joint planning and collaboration between local agencies with the production of joint plans a key requirement.

At a national level, Griffiths is critical of central government's ambivalence and procrastination over community care for the past 30 years or so. He put forward a number of proposals to give a sharper focus to policy in this area. Above all, he is emphatic that over-ambitious policy goals should not be established without sufficient resources to meet them. He also excluded major structural reform believing that 'nothing could be more radical in the public sector than to spell out responsibilities, insist on performance and accountability and to evidence that action is being taken; and even more radical, to match policy with appropriate resources and agreed timescales' (para 20). As if anticipating subsequent events, Griffiths warned that his proposals were to be taken as a whole 'and no single one on its own'. In his view, 'merely to tinker with the present system would not address the central issues and would forego the benefits that could be obtained from more concentrated action'.

Finally, Griffiths was acutely aware of the rapid pace of change and of the danger of offering solutions which were inappropriate to changed circumstances. We return to this concern in the next section.

Despite a general consensus across the political spectrum in support of Griffiths' diagnosis and prescription, the government did not respond to the report for over a year. There was much in the report which the government disliked, particularly Griffiths' insistence on the lead role for SSDs, and on the need for central government to be clear about its policy objectives and to match these with the resources needed to meet them. For a government which made no attempt to conceal its dislike of local government nor wished to be explicit about policies and objectives for fear of being held responsible for their failure and inadequate resourcing, the Griffiths prescription proved especially unpleasant to swallow. A further cause of the delay in responding to the Griffiths report was the government's growing preoccupation with the NHS following a review which had taken most of 1988 to complete. A White Paper on the NHS appeared in 1989 accompanied by considerable publicity. As ever, health services (especially the acute sector) absorbed Ministers' attention and community care remained something of a policy backwater. With the implementation of the NHS reforms in April 1991, they have continued to occupy centre stage.

Growing pressure on the government to make some response to Griffiths, coupled with an awareness that many of the NHS reforms depended for their success on getting community care sorted out, finally obliged the Secretary of State for Health to act. Consequently, a statement was given to Parliament in July 1989 which served as a sort of holding operation, or *hors d'oeuvres* to the main course – the White Paper – which eventually appeared in November 1989. Its appearance was low key, in striking contrast to the arrival of the NHS White Paper some 10 months earlier.

The proposals contained in the White Paper, *Caring for People*, followed the main thrust of the Griffiths agenda. The central objective was to enable people to be cared for and remain in their own homes supported as necessary to do so. New financial arrangements were to be introduced to remove the perverse incentive towards residential or nursing home care – responsibilities were to be clarified and local authorities were to assume primary responsibility for 'assessing individual need, designing care arrangements and securing their delivery within available resources'. Ministers reluctantly adopted Griffiths' preference for the enabling role to be performed by local government but only after rejecting the alternatives and in a manner betraying sufficient lack of conviction to suggest that further change could not be excluded. Where the White Paper and the Griffiths report diverged most sharply was in respect of finance and central government's responsibilities. On finance, the government rejected the proposal for a specific grant for community care (with the exception of the modest specific grant for mental illness services) opting instead to channel resources via the general Revenue Support Grant. In transferring resources in this way, community care would take its place among other local authority priorities with no certainty that resources transferred would find their way into community care. In regard to central government, the view taken was that the Department of Health was already doing all it could to facilitate and create the conditions and incentives for successful policy implementation.

After the White Paper

Although flawed in a number of important respects, not least of these being the continuing uncertainty about the future of long-term care in the NHS as distinct from local authorities, the view among observers was that although the White Paper was an ill-conceived and hastily assembled document, it at least ended several years of uncertainty and virtual 'planning blight'. The waiting had ended. Or so it was believed.

But nearly a year after his first statement to Parliament on the community care reforms, the Secretary of State for Health gave a further statement announcing a delay and a phasing in of the reforms. Whereas the original intention had been to implement the changes on 1 April 1991 alongside the NHS reforms, the government decided that its political fortunes over the Community Charge, or poll tax, were sufficiently precarious to warrant a delay in implementing the community care changes. Under the revised timetable, implementation is being phased over three years starting in April 1991 and ending in April 1993. The details are given in Table 2

The delay over implementation, together with more recent developments in respect of local government finance, functions and structure, have fuelled anxieties about the government's commitment to community care in general and to a local government lead role in particular. While policy and practice guidance continues to appear and Ministers continue

Table 2. *Phased implementation*

Stage 1: April 1991
Financial
- new Specific Grant for Mental Illness
- new Specific Grant for Drugs and Alcohol

Implementation
- setting up inspection units
- setting up complaints procedures
- work to develop and implement the 'purchaser–provider' split

Developmental
- work on local authority and health authority plans
- continue with general development projects

Stage 2: April 1992
Implementation
- local authority and health authority plans

Developmental
- test out proposals on assessment/care management in preparation for the transfer of the care element of social security funding

Stage 3: April 1993
Financial
- transfer of social security for new cases after April 1993
- introduction of assessment and care management procedures

Source: Henwood, Jowell & Wistow (1991)

to give assurances that implementation is going ahead, there is a sense in which moves like this may be compared to rearranging the deck-chairs on the Titanic. What is the point of all these tactical manoeuvres if the policy itself looks increasingly precarious? After all, the issue is not *whether* local government will remain in its present form but rather *what* its future shape will be.

If only because 1993 is a long way off for any government, there must be doubt over whether a coherent policy can be said to exist in respect of community care – if it ever did. With an election in the offing and with both major political parties committed to a review of local government, albeit for different reasons, there is considerable uncertainty over whether the current reform agenda will ever see the light of day. In the meantime, the perverse incentive whereby health and local authorities access the care element of the social security budget in order to fund residential care and nursing home care in the private sector for elderly people remains intact. As various studies have demonstrated, it is arguable whether such care is the most appropriate for many of these who find their way into it. Although the reform proposals are designed to address the problem, this will not happen until the transfer of resources from the social security budget takes place in 1993 (Henwood, Jowell & Wistow 1991). The immediate future heralds no great change in respect of policy on long-term care. Such care will, for better or worse, continue for the most part to take place in residential care settings in the private sector.

In the longer run, the intention is to develop domiciliary based services and retain residential care for those assessed as being in need of it. Issues will then begin to arise over whose responsibility it is to provide long-term care for elderly people. Indeed, they have aleady surfaced, with no clear policy apparent from the centre to guide decisions. Policy in this area is being left to the local agencies to agree. The health service may well consider that long-term care is no longer its responsibility and should reside with local authorities. On the other hand, local authorities may feel that if there is a health care component then the health service should at least make some contribution to the continuing care of such service users. The health/social care divide is a very real one although it makes little sense to those elderly people whose needs transcend that boundary. There is a distinct possibility of an emerging 'care gap' and increasingly fragmented services.

Another consequence of the reforms is the potential for acute sector bed blocking by elderly people who are unable to be discharged into the community because of a lack of adequate support. For local authorities the priority is likely to be people already residing in the community in need of support rather than those who will be discharged from hospital. The whole future of joint planning between health and social services could be put in jeopardy if there is a breakdown or absence of dialogue between these two agencies and a continuation of the distrust and mutual suspicion which has characterised much of what passes for joint planning (Hunter & Richards 1990, Hunter & Wistow 1991).

For these and related reasons, many observers and policy-makers have begun to cast around for other solutions which do not depend upon local government at a time of probable upheaval. This provides the perfect excuse for those who never really approved of the policy and who would rather see, for instance, the NHS assume total responsibility for community care. There are those who believe the NHS is both more committed to community care than local government and does it better.

At the time of writing the state of policy-making in respect of community care remains confused and unstable. Despite attempts to resolve a number of central concerns they remain unresolved. In particular, it remains unclear whether the White Paper changes, enshrined in the 1990

Act, will take root or whether they will be replaced, at least partially, by a new policy which is yet to be fashioned. But whatever else, the changes now being contemplated will not in themselves be sufficient to address the longer term needs of elderly people over the next decade.

The longer term

What about the longer term in respect of social care for elderly people? Sir Roy Griffiths in his review of community care said:

I have the occasional sinking feeling that there is nothing so outdated as to provide today's solution to today's problem. There is a need to experiment with a whole variety of initiatives.

Sir Roy's observation echoes some of the arguments advanced in the government's most recent policy statement on elderly people, *Growing Older* (DHSS 1981). This White Paper emphasised that the role of the State in meeting the needs of elderly people will have to change to 'an enabling one, helping people to care for themselves and their families' (para 6.10). It is argued that the public expenditure implications of maintaining existing policies and standards of public provision are so considerable that radical changes in the development of social policy are in need of urgent consideration. This is principally because,

The increasing needs of increasing numbers of older people simply cannot be met wholly – or even predominantly – by public authorities or public finance. This will be a task for the whole community, demanding the closest partnership between public and voluntary bodies, families and individuals. The framework of cooperation has to be developed now.   *(para 9.6)*

There are a number of ways of responding to this injunction and Griffiths does no more than indicate the possibilities in very general terms. These include: social/health maintainance organisations and other forms of social care insurance. He also suggests that corporate financial planning in future years may reflect growing concern about community care in the way that support for occupational pensions developed after the Second World War. But there may also be a case for action to be taken by government to lead the way. Griffiths suggests the following:

More immediately there is no reason why, on a controlled basis, social services authorities should not experiment with vouchers or credits for particular levels of community care, allowing individuals to spend them on particular forms of domiciliary care and to choose between particular suppliers as they wish.

(para 39)

This final section focuses on long-term care funding and on options for social care insurance because in the UK this market is poised to take off. It has already done so in some European countries, notably Germany, and also in the United States. The results in these countries have been mixed and we have much to learn from the early experience of long-term care insurance. The chief issues centre on demographic changes, the wealth of elderly people, and the attitudes of institutional investors. As was pointed out in the first section above, the ageing of the population, together with an increase in the need for care among the rising numbers of those aged 85 and over, constitutes the context in which long-term care policy will be shaped.

The chief reason for growing interest in long-term insurance is a very simple one, namely, the alleged growing affluence of elderly people. In the jargon, they are asset rich, income poor. There is increasing talk of 'Woopies' (Well Off Older People) and 'Jollies' (Jet-setting Oldies with Lots of Loot). By the end of the century some 65–70% of elderly house-holders will be owner occupiers. But although some older people will be more affluent, spending money on care services is likely to be a low priority for them (Sinclair *et al.*, 1990). Moreover, developments in occupational pensions and schemes to release equity in housing are unlikely to make sufficient resources available for care (Sinclair *et al.*, 1990).

With an ageing population giving cause for concern about the pressure on public expenditure and its ability to cope, as it is beginning to do, shifting the responsibility onto insurance and onto private sources of finance looks increasingly attractive in theory. But what of the reality? As Phillips (1989) observes, available data for 1988 show that the income of elderly people is really very low (see Table 3), with 98% of people then aged 85 + having incomes of £200 per week or less. The same income level applied to 86% of people aged 61–70 years. 'The point to emphasise, therefore, is that income levels fall among the mass of the population as they get older' (p. 33). Even in respect of elderly people with occupational pensions, 78% have incomes under £200 a week. 'Very few people aged 70 and over have more than £20 000 a year' (*ibid*). Sinclair and his colleagues (1990) confirm this position, pointing out that 'a substantial proportion, probably half, of all retirement pensioners live in poverty (defined as below 140% of income support scale rates). They tend to become poorer as they get older and it is amongst older elderly people that needs accumulate. Clearly this large group has virtually no prospect of purchasing private care' (p. 63). The researchers estimate that possibly as few as 10% of all elderly households could purchase private care services in their

Table 3. *National average family income data by age*

		% Age Groups (Years)				
Income £	Nat Av.	41–50	51–60	61–70	71–80	85 +
Nil – 4500	28	10	20	51	70	83
4500– 9500	29	26	34	35	24	15
9500–13 500	17	20	17	7	4	2
13 500–17 500	11	16	12	4	1	–
17 500 +	15	28	17	3	1	–

Source: Financial Research Services 1988 (quoted in Phillips 1989)

own homes on a regular basis. Financing care from savings on a large scale is not therefore a viable option.

The scope for financing care from assets and equity locked up in housing is a more likely prospect, although not without limitations, and is therefore an important area for consideration. Insurance based opportunities could therefore appear more attractive although it should not be overlooked that the need for continued public funding is unavoidable whatever policy instruments are favoured. Nevertheless, the longer term position is one in which an increasing number of people will be able to insure against their future social care needs should they wish to do so.

If this is so, then it is surprising that the government has not included any mention of insurance in its plans for community care or long-term care in general. Tax incentives will be necessary to encourage long-term care insurance on a sizeable scale. In this respect, government policy and a benign attitude on the part of central government to long-term care insurance will also be necessary. In the NHS reforms there is the commitment to allow tax relief for people aged 65 and over to enable them and/or their carers to take out private health insurance. This sets a precedent in the way in which health services in the UK are funded and is potentially a significant move in respect of the future funding of long-term care and the development of insurance schemes for this sector. Few, however, expect this specific proposal to have much impact in itself on the financing and availability of care for older people.

Long-term care insurance is not, of course, without its problems. A key one is the coverage restrictions associated with it. For example, certain age groups (i.e. 85 and over) may be excluded from coverage as well as those suffering from certain conditions, i.e. Alzheimer's disease and other forms of dementia. If such restrictions are removed, as has occurred in respect of second generation insurance products, it is at the cost of high premiums thereby reducing the number of elderly people who can afford them.

To summarise, long-term care insurance carries with it three critical limitations:

policies are not sold to people who are very old or chronically impaired

benefits may be specified in fixed sterling terms which means that individuals may pay premiums for cover which may be far from adequate when the time comes for that cover to be taken up if the inflation rate has in the interim eroded the available cover

premiums can be raised at will by companies with the result that cover may be insufficient for the purposes for which it was originally purchased.

Long-term care insurance may be a more attractive option through employment rather than through individuals. But companies' willingness to shoulder the cost of long-term insurance or any proportion of it seems unlikely. Already, companies are complaining about the amount they are expected to do to substitute for state welfare and contributing to the long-term care of elderly people would probably be rejected as being unacceptably burdensome. Private long-term insurance, then, seems likely to fall short of what is needed. At the end of the day, it is unlikely to afford adequate protection.

What about social insurance as an option to finance long-term care for elderly people? This has the attraction of spreading the risk over the largest population and over time, and insures the already impaired as well as the healthy while allowing for an equitable distribution of burdens and costs across income groups. The virtue of a social insurance scheme is that it would allow funds to be explicitly identified and earmarked for long-term care purposes. Under the present system of public funding this degree of explicitness is not possible. Yet, people of all ages and income groups may be willing to pay the price for long-term care if it can be made explicit and identifiable through some form of social insurance. However, such a development is unlikely without considerable assistance from government through tax and other incentives. But the costs will be high and whether the government is prepared to shoulder these is by no means certain. Similar problems are already being encountered in respect of services funded from general taxation.

The notion of social/health maintenance organisations proposed by Griffiths and others (e.g. for a discussion of BRITSMOS see Davies and

Challis 1986) is an innovative approach to the financing and organisation of care for elderly people based on the Health Maintenance Organization (HMO) concept in the US. HMOs operate on a capitation arrangement, with patients enrolled on an annual basis for a set fee and guaranteed comprehensive medical care. The HMO provides for all their primary and acute medical needs at no further charge. HMOs may be hospitals, hospital-based, or free-standing facilities that contract with local hospitals for in-patient care. HMOs can employ doctors and other staff on a fixed salary basis or, alternatively, doctors in independent practices can form an association and be paid a set amount to manage each patient. The incentive in an HMO is to keep patients as healthy as possible since profit is dependent on spending less for care than on total subscriptions. Some HMOs have demonstrated that they can provide care at 10–40% less than the cost of comparable care in a fee-for-service setting. The proposed social maintenance organisation would adapt the basic concept to deal with long-term dependency in elderly people. It would operate a case management system and essentially perform a 'brokerage function' by negotiating with existing providers to obtain access to, and the lowest cost services for, its members. Although proposed experiments with such a model have been put forward, none has yet been established. Nevertheless, the idea has attracted considerable interest from various quarters, including financial institutions.

Concluding comment

The lessons for future policy for the financing and provision of long-term care are unclear. Present policy remains muddled, confused and unstable. There is a need for good policy analysis. Regrettably, it is notably lacking within government. As Phillips (1989) notes, 'insuring old age is a highly complex subject, ... (about which) there is hardly any experience worldwide' (p. 35). Although 1.3 million long-term care policies are in force in the USA, more than 85% of them are three years old or less. Such impressive growth, however, does not reveal much about the optimum approach given the limited experience to date. Two key problems are the extent to which poor people are excluded or can only afford inadequate cover, and the fact that people in work do not want to think much beyond their retirement income requirements. They do not attach priority to long-term social care needs.

We cannot ignore the fact that for all the talk of rising prosperity and affluence among elderly people there remain considerable inequalities in

old age. As noted earlier, the new affluence among older people has
touched only a minority albeit a sizeable one. Most older people live on
low incomes and have few assets. Even home ownership gives rise to
major inequalities in respect of the quality and cost of housing. It should
be remembered that almost 30% of households in which the head is aged
75 and over have incomes in the lowest 10% of income distribution and
almost three-quarters fall within the lowest 30%. No other age group is so
heavily represented at the lower end of income distribution. This position
will not change much in the foreseeable future.

All community care policies contain contradictions (Sinclair *et al.*,
1990). Present policy is no exception and conceals a number of implicit
conflicts and ambivalences. These include: the wish to increase resources
for care by encouraging the private sector and the wish to distribute these
resources according to need; between the virtues of innovation and
competition and the need for equity and comprehensiveness in the supply
of community care; and between a professional assessment of need as a
means of accessing resources and the desire to encourage consumer
choice. Assuming that there is a commitment to establishing a coherent
policy framework for long-term care for elderly people, five principles
may be established in underpinning such a policy. They are:

achieving a balance between public and private finance

ensuring that a concern with cost containment does not lead to an
underfunding of benefits

ensuring that a concern with fiscal fairness across population groups
and generations does not undermine the commitment to pool resources
to help those who are unable to help themselves

avoiding service fragmentation as the delivery of care becomes more
pluralistic and attractive to new independent sector suppliers

thinking of long-term care not as a problem, i.e. as part of the burden of
dependency thesis all too often associated with old age, but as an
opportunity to enable old people to lead satisfying and fulfilling lives.

If much of the content of this chapter has appeared somewhat negative
and gives cause for concern about the potential for future policy in
long-term care and its likely direction there are no apologies to be made.
Until we address long-term care policy for elderly people in hard-headed
terms both in respect of its funding and its provision it is unlikely that we
will do anything other than continue to mouth empty rhetoric and muddle
along. But there is a glimmer of light and hope for the future. We should

not underestimate the power of elderly people as a political force for real change. The force has yet to be organised and to make much impact on the political scene. But the potential is there for it to do so and there is evidence from the United States that this will indeed be the case. Those people currently in their late seventies and eighties have grown up in an era when deference to authority was acceptable and a questioning of services and benefits received was considered unreasonable. This cohort effect will gradually wither away as people entering their later years have little experience of anything other than public welfare services established after the war. These groups represent a force for change in respect of policies and practices for those in need of long-term care. They are our best hope for improving policy in an area which has singularly lacked imagination and sustained commitment from successive governments.

References

Audit Commission (1986), *Making a Reality of Community Care*, London: HMSO.

Davies, B. & Challis, D. (1986). *Matching Resources to Needs in Community Care*, Aldershot: Gower.

Department of Health and Social Security (1981), *Growing Older*, London: HMSO.

Griffiths, Sir Roy (1988). *Community Care: Agenda for Action*, London: HMSO.

Henwood, M. (1990). *Community Care and Elderly People*, London: Family Policy Studies Centre.

Henwood, M. Jowell, T. & Wistow, G. (1991). *All Things Come (To those Who Wait?)* Briefing Paper 12, London: King's Fund Institute, Joseph Rowntree Foundation, Nuffield Institute for Health Services Studies.

Hunter, D. J. & Judge, K. (1988). *Griffiths and Community Care: Meeting the Challenge*, Briefing Paper 5, London: King's Fund Institute.

Hunter, D. J. & Richards, H. (1990). *Towards a Framework for Joint Planning in Scotland*, Central Research Unit Papers, Edinburgh: Scottish Office.

Hunter, D. J. & Wistow, G. (eds) (1989). *Principles and Responsibilities in Community Care*, Leeds: Nuffield Institute for Health Services Studies.

Hunter, D. J. & Wistow, G. (1991). *Elderly People's Integrated Care System (EPICS): An Organisational, Policy and Practice Review*, Nuffield Institute Reports No. 3, Leeds: Nuffield Institute for Health Services Studies.

Phillips, M. (1989). 'The Independent Sector'. In Hunter and Wistow (eds), *op. cit.*

Sinclair, I. Parker, R. Leat, D. & Williams, J. (1990). *The Kaleidescope of Care*, National Institute for Social Work, London: HMSO.

World Health Organisation (1989). *Health of the Elderly*, Technical Report Series 779, Geneva: WHO.

10

What is required for good quality in long-term care of the elderly?

MARION HILDICK-SMITH

Public attitudes to the old must change. We must stop devaluing them and forgetting their past and present contribution to society. Only then will there be the readiness to fund the long-term care they may need. Many elderly people are able to support themselves. They may have benefited from the increased value of their homes, or been able to contribute to an occupational pension; they may be in good health and have family or friends nearby. However, others, through no fault of their own, may be in a quite different situation. They may have cared for relatives instead of going out to work, or alternatively may have worked in low-paid jobs and been unable to save. They may suffer from increasing physical or mental disability beyond the capacity of their carers. They may live far from any relatives or may have outlived their families. They are a vulnerable group and could easily be exploited when they need long-term care if there are not adequate safeguards.

Both within the health service and in the growing private and voluntary sector there is great variation between the best and worst types of long-term care. As the number of hospital long-stay beds has diminished, research in our unit has shown that the physical dependency of our remaining long-stay patients has increased, and their mental capability diminished. This change must be mirrored in increased staffing levels otherwise standards in hospital long-term care will worsen. The somewhat-less-disabled patients are now cared for in many areas in nursing homes whose standards and staffing are subject to inspection by nurses from the district health authority. Residential homes are inspected by the local authority and are not meant to take people who need continuous nursing care unless they have dual registration. Some residential homes provide a very good standard of care. Others often have vacancies, and proprietors may ring up the hospital offering to take patients who, in our view, are beyond their capacity to care for properly. They may not have the staff or equipment to look after those who need physical nursing care, nor the knowledge and training to help patients who, for example, are prone to behave in an agitated or disturbed fashion.

Much long-term care of the elderly takes place within the community, as many severely handicapped people are cared for by their families. There is increasing recognition of the role of the carers, and the proposals for community care must include adequate community support services and opportunity for respite care. In our own unit up to 14 patients, who would otherwise have been cared for in long-term hospital beds, are managed at home by their carers helped by nurses visiting two or three times daily. The nurses were funded out of savings from the closure of a 14-bed hospital ward. It has proved possible to care for even very heavily dependent patients by this means, provided there is a carer at home, and provided the patient is rational enough to appreciate being at home. Respite care in a nearby long-stay geriatric ward, say for 2 weeks in each 3 months, enables many carers to carry on so that their relative eventually dies at home, as was their wish.

On the other hand, many patients, for a variety of reasons, have to spend their last months or years in an institution, and much of our effort is directed at making this as satisfactory a substitute for home as possible. There is no lack of guidance on good practices in long-term care, for example in 'Home Life' (1984) or the booklet 'Improving Care of Elderly People in Hospital' (1987). This latter document was published by the Royal College of Nursing in association with the British Geriatrics Society and the Royal College of Psychiatrists. The Health Advisory Service gives examples of good practices which are found, for example, in long-term wards during its visits to geriatric and psychogeriatric services all over the country. A new report will soon be published on 'Good practice in long-term care' initiated by the Royal College of Physicians' Research Unit. Members of the working party who produced the report included representatives from the British Geriatrics Society and the Royal College of Psychiatrists, together with an ethicist and an elderly home resident. The guidelines are not difficult to define, and the problem is not that of defining them, but of trying to achieve them in the face of staffing difficulties and poor buildings.

A central issue is that of nurse staffing, training and attitudes. We owe a great deal to dedicated nurses and care staff who show love and understanding even of the most difficult and demanding of their patients. They find satisfaction in small improvements in patients' capabilities, and can be a great support to patients and relatives at times of deterioration and death. Nurse attitudes and morale were greatly helped in long-stay units around the country by the discussions which took place using the training slides associated with the first booklet 'Improving Geriatric Care in Hospital' in 1975. Subjects such as 'personal dignity and privacy' or 'terminal care' gave rise in our unit to lively discussions between many different staff members – from doctors, nurses, therapists and social workers to porters, ambulancemen and chaplains. We all gained in knowledge of the subject and of each others' points of view. Morale improved and it was a pleasure to see how many staff were willing to attend during off-duty time. The exercise was repeated twice since, partly because staff had changed, and it will probably need to be repeated again after the present upheavals in the hospital service have settled down. Nurses skilled in long-term care are a scarce resource, so it is important that only those patients who have been fully assessed and have had the chance of rehabilitation should be deemed to need long-term nursing and medical care. Such multidisciplinary assessment was the rule when long-term care was within the hospital sector and under consultant supervision. It will be difficult to achieve if patients are admitted to different homes and under different general practitioners. For those who will be paid for from public funds it seems reasonable to assess first whether treatment or rehabilitation would obviate the need for long-term support. This assessment needs the skills of a multidisciplinary team with a consultant geriatrician or psychogeriatrician, or other doctor trained in geriatric medicine. It is a complex and time-consuming task to ensure that a patient, often ill or at a crisis in her life, has every opportunity to improve or adapt before moving into an institution, perhaps for the rest of her days.

Assessment is not only important on entry into long-term care. Reassessment at intervals is also of value in showing whether there has been improvement or deterioration, and whether further benefit can be achieved. In a study comparing hospital long-stay wards with NHS nursing homes (Bond *et al.* 1989) 11% of patients were discharged from hospital long-stay wards when they no longer needed the level of care provided. However only 1% of patients were discharged from the NHS nursing homes (where they could stay even if they improved). The hospital long-stay wards were more efficient at rationing the expensive resource, but the NHS nursing home was allowing the patients freedom to choose to stay – and the two aims are clearly in conflict.

Periodic reassessment is also of importance to patients because other remediable conditions may arise and be treated. However this type of structured review is unlikely to occur when long-term care patients are under the care of a general practitioner in a number of different nursing homes. There is a danger that medical support will be episodic and in response to crisis, and that there will be little incentive for continued rehabilitation or for auditing of standards.

Audit measures must take account of the ways in which old people are different from younger ones. Diseases present atypically in old people and may be compounded by the fact that the patient has several diseases at once. The elderly patient may have poor physical reserves, so that a further minor illness is the last straw. Similarly because of poor mental reserves an elderly patient may more easily become confused because of an infection or operation. Great care is needed in the number and dosage of drugs given to ill elderly people because of these poor physical and mental reserves. Good training in all these aspects is essential for staff in long-term care. In addition they need to have detailed knowledge of some common problems.

They need to know how to prevent urinary incontinence by having patients up and dressed in day clothes, by regular toileting, by having a bedside commode at night and by having lavatories within easy walking distance of dayrooms. They need to be alert to investigate newly-occurring incontinence. They need to be well-informed about incontinence pads and to insist on being supplied with ones of good quality. With good nursing attention faecal incontinence can be reduced from an average of 50% in all types of long-term care to about 5%. This can be done by clearing the bowel with enemas and preventing recurrence of constipation by a combination of diet, fluids, stool-bulking agents and bowel training.

Half of those aged 75 and over fall in the course of a year, and about half of these falls occur in institutions. They have multiple causes – poor vision, poor balance, mental confusion, poor staffing levels, poor lighting, and some of these can be tackled. The risk of falls in the elderly must be balanced against a reasonable degree of autonomy for the elderly themselves. This is often difficult, and the help and advice of physiotherapists can be very valuable, and supportive to the nurses.

Psychological aspects of nursing care are also important, displayed, for example, in encouraging dependent patients to do more for themselves, or in recognising when a patient is becoming depressed. In psychogeriatric long-term care the problems of the wandering patient must be addressed together with those of patients with paranoid or disturbed behaviour. Well trained and understanding nurses can help these patients in a kind and gentle manner using techniques of distraction instead of resorting to over sedation. Similar measures will help agitated or confused patients and good support from medical staff is needed. Clear medical records are vital and must include a test of mental score together with assessment of vision or hearing or capacity for communication.

Staff in other hospital departments also need training, as is suggested, for example, by the fact that most pressure sores develop in casualty or X-ray or theatre and could be prevented if staff ensured that all patients lay on supportive mattresses on the hospital trollies. Once such a sore has developed it can take many weeks and be very costly to heal. Prevention and treatment of all the physical and psychological problems I have mentioned can restore to patients their sense of dignity and self-respect, and improve their morale so that they can achieve their maximum potential.

As people get older they are more likely to be susceptible to adverse drug reactions, yet it is precisely the most susceptible group, the frail over 75 group, who will be receiving medication in long-term care wards. Polypharmacy should be avoided whenever possible. Regular review of therapy, with the aim of stopping unnecessary drugs, is an important part of good practice. Use of sedatives and tranquillisers can be kept to a minimum when staff are well trained and supervised. There is little information about use of drugs in nursing homes. However the level of prescriptions was high in one study in nursing homes in Weston-super-Mare (Hepple *et al.* 1989) and poor medical records were being kept. More research is needed into how long-term units (both hospitals and homes) tackle the problems of medication in frail elderly people who have a number of different diseases. The Royal College of Physicians' working party will suggest audit measures for medication. These will be piloted to make sure they are well-selected and not too time-consuming in use. If they are found useful in practice their general use could be recommended.

An important indicator of good quality long-term care is the level of care given to the dying patient. Hospital long-term wards have gained greatly from the advances in this field, pioneered by workers in the hospice movement. There is much greater openness now in discussing matters of life and death with patients and relatives and getting to know their views. A complicating factor in geriatric long-term care is that many of the patients, in addition to their severe physical incapacity, suffer from increasing degrees of dementia. Despite all efforts their quality of life is often very poor. It can be very helpful if relatives and staff can discuss, in an individual case, whether the time has come when efforts to prolong life are no longer appropriate. Relatives may shy away from stating too definite views, and the issue needs to be approached sensitively. It may be clear that further treatment is burdensome for the patient, or that its effect is to prolong the act of dying. As a Christian I find the comments of a Church of England working party in 1975 helpful. They said that 'Extraordinary means of treatment should not be used for the terminally ill', also that 'Treatment can be used to relieve pain that may shorten life'. This does not, of course, imply any reduction of care, rather the reverse. Any condition or symptom which may distress the patient must be treated, all nursing care given, together with whatever psychological support is necessary for patients and relatives. Other patients, too, may need help to cope with the death of one of their number – both to grieve and to face the possibility of their own death. For doctors in long-term care it is increasingly important to recognise pre-death and to know when to change from so-called 'aggressive' treatment to 'palliative' treatment. Life and death are in God's hands and it is up to us to use our skills and experience as best we can, and to recognise that our powers are more limited than we, or our patients, think. Decisions are often difficult and there may not be a 'right' view, only a less wrong one.

Patients' views are not only needed on life and death issues, but also in day-to-day matters. They need choice of what to eat and what to wear, whether to be in company or to spend some time alone or in quietness. Some will be happy talking over old photographs in a reminiscence corner, others will be happier with a book in a quiet room. For some television is companionship and liveliness – for others it is intrusive and irrelevant. Neither television nor radio should be constantly on nor tuned to programmes for the benefit of the staff.

Much long-term care is given in old and unsuitable buildings with poor equipment, and insufficient toilets and bathrooms. There is little privacy for those who want it. However some patients prefer the activity of a shared living-space and would not want to be 'shut away' in a single room, especially if staff are few and there is little chance of visitors. Old buildings may make it very difficult for the patients to have an acceptable choice in this matter. Private homes have placed more value on privacy, and there is a welcome tendency to provide each patient with her own toilet, which adds greatly to an individual's sense of dignity and privacy.

Not long ago, on behalf of the Royal Surgical Aids Society, I visited a number of recently-built homes with two architect colleagues. We were judging a competition to find the winning home which provided complete care for the elderly and was of architectural merit. It was encouraging to see how local and housing authorities, charities and private organisations and the health service could build well for the elderly. One of the features of the good designs was the mixture of public and private spaces, bustling and quiet rooms, allowing variety and choice. Many had design features which would enable elderly and handicapped people to maintain their maximum independence. Some had taken advice from staff working in homes and institutions, or had gradually improved on the variant of the design which was first built in previous years by incorporating suggestions from staff and residents. We particularly looked for homes which would be able to keep their residents even when they deteriorated. Moving into an institution is traumatic in old age, and it seems better to bring increased help to the resident in the home rather than expecting residents to move repeatedly as they worsen.

Although the winning designs were not the most expensive of those submitted, cost is clearly a limiting factor in designing for long-term care and in revenue needed to run the units. Some of the expansion of private homes over the last 10 years has been fuelled by the financial arrangements (see the previous chapter by Hunter). These provide a 'perverse incentive' for people to go into homes rather than continue to manage at home with community services. Present Government policy (*Caring for People* 1989) is to reverse this trend and encourage more people to be supported at home. This policy, if and when it is properly funded, has the strong support of the British Geriatrics Society. However for those who do need institutional long-term care appropriate funding and staffing will be required. Many of these elderly people have contributed greatly to society in earlier years. We must strive to improve the conditions in which they live in long-term care so that they can have some of the choices we take for granted in our everyday lives.

References

Bond, J., Gregson, B. A. & Atkinson, A. (1989). Measurement of outcomes within a multicentred randomised controlled trial in the evaluation of the experimental NHS nursing homes. *Age and Ageing*, **18**, 292–302.

Caring for People. Community care in the next decade and beyond. 1989 London. HMSO.

Hepple, J., Bowler, I. & Bowman, C. E. (1989). A survey of private nursing home residents in Weston-super-Mare. *Age and Ageing*, **18**, 61–3.

Home Life (1984). A code of practice for residential care. Report of a working party sponsored by the DHSS and convened by the Centre for Policy on Aging.

Improving Geriatric Care in Hospital (1975). Royal College of Nursing.

Improving Care of Elderly People in Hospital (1987). Royal College of Nursing, Ruislip Press.

11

Should age make a difference in health care entitlement?

JOSEPH BOYLE

The health care needed by many people, not only by the elderly, is limited for a variety of reasons. Sometimes a person does not want certain medical treatments, and it is often reasonable and morally correct for one to act on such a desire; sometimes others decide not to provide health care for a patient not capable of deciding for himself or herself, because of their judgment that such treatment does not help the patient or harms the patient more than it helps him or her. But sometimes health care is limited, not out of concern for patients' well-being or legitimate desires, but because there are not sufficient resources to provide the needed care. The moral issues raised by these different grounds for limiting health care are distinct, although, as I will suggest, they are sometimes confused. I will be focusing only on limitations based on the scarcity of health care resources.

A scarcity of health care resources can emerge within any social arrangement for providing health care. Perhaps the most obvious situations in which this happens are medical disasters when triage is called for to distribute fairly resources which, in the circumstances, are insufficient to assist all who need them. But such situations can also arise when families have the responsibility for the health care of their members and lack the money and other resources both to provide the needed care and to fulfill other exigent obligations. And they can also arise within systems in which there are health care entitlements, that is, in societies where the government provides or pays for some or all of the health care of citizens and residents.

It is clear that one of the reasons why health care is provided or paid for by the government is that societies have greater resources than individuals or families for meeting health care needs. This suggests that something has gone very wrong if the health care provided to people by a system of

147

entitlements is not better than they could provide, and would feel duty bound to provide, for themselves and others without such a system. But the relatively greater resources of a society should not lead to the expectation that there will be *no* limits to health care entitlements.

Indeed, the conjunction of two undeniable facts implies that there must be some limits on the health care to which people are entitled. First, the overall resources of any society are finite and must be used to support a variety of socially important activities such as education, transportation and communication, and police and defense, as well as a variety of health care services. Second, the demands for health care are open ended and capable of indefinite expansion. Anyone who is helped to recover a level of good health by one set of medical interventions may have reason to seek a more satisfactory level of health, and will probably get sick again in the future. It is clear that the predicament generated by these facts exists today in countries like the United Kingdom, Canada and the United States. Health care costs are increasing as a proportion of the overall expenditures of these countries, and there is widespread discussion of how to contain these costs, as well as concern about the impact of the level of health care spending on other social services.

So, health care entitlements have to be limited because even wealthy societies lack the resources for providing all the health care which people have reason to seek. Furthermore, this limitation is plainly of a kind which requires several types of social choice. First, social choices are required to determine how much of a society's resources are to be devoted to health care. Secondly, social choices are needed to determine priorities within health care. Since there are many kinds of help a health care system can provide – preventive medicine, basic entry level diagnosis and treatment, acute care, and so on – and since the resources available for health care are limited, we must decide which kinds of health care to provide and at what levels. Thirdly, further social choices are needed within the framework established by the first two kinds of choice in order to determine fairly who is to receive health care benefits when situations of scarcity arise with the effect that not all who need them can be helped. However social choices of the first two kinds are settled, modern health care has, and as a practical matter is bound to have, resources – such things as procedures, personnel and equipment – which can be used to help some but not all who need them. So choices are needed about who is to receive and who is to be denied such benefits.

For convenience, I will call choices of the first two kinds 'allocation decisions' and those of the third kind 'rationing decisions.' In making this distinction, I am not seeking to obscure the complex interrelations between what I call allocation decisions and rationing decisions, nor am I suggesting that all social decisions about distributing health care benefits can be neatly classified into one of these categories. I make the distinction only because the moral issues raised by allocation decisions are somewhat different from those raised by rationing decisions.

It seems clear that neither allocation nor rationing decisions can be morally good unless they are in accord with principles of social justice and simple fairness. But the implications of the requirements of social justice and fairness with respect to allocation decisions within a society having a system of health care entitlements are often obscure. This obscurity is rooted in the difficulty of elaborating the moral foundation of health care entitlements and of entitlements generally.

My own account of this matter is as follows: the extent of health care entitlements substantially depends upon the personal, familial and neigh-bourly obligations which each of us has towards health; and the concrete, practical implications of these obligations are contingent upon a variety of factors such as our overall resources and other obligations. What we are morally bound to do to help others at this pre-institutional level provides at least a rough indicator (and surely the minimum level) of what we are obliged to provide for others within our society by supporting the system of health care entitlements. For the moral foundation of a system of health care entitlements is that such a system implements and facilitates our carrying out of these common human obligations concerning our own and others' health care.[1]

The other accounts of the moral foundations of health care entitle-ments of which I am aware do not reduce the indeterminacies which my account acknowledges. Consequently, allocation decisions are bound to be morally complex.

By way of contrast, the moral assessment of rationing decisions is more straightforward because very frequently the only moral issue in these choices is whether or not they are fair in providing needed help to some and denying it to others. Those who must make these decisions face them because of the discrepancy between need and available resources which remains after health care and other social priorities have been established, and which cannot be avoided by future changes in policy. Thus, the situations calling for rationing decisions often eliminate the relevance of any moral considerations besides those of fairness in dealing with those who have some claim on the scarce resources.

Consider, for example, a hospital which has only a given number of intensive care beds, and in which the demand for those beds at a given time exceeds the number available. Even if the hospital authorities rightly believe that more beds are required, they must decide which patients among all who need their use are to be permitted to use them. A reconsideration of established allocation decisions may be morally called for, and unjust allocation decisions may be among the causes of the situation, but a rationing decision is unavoidable. Clearly, such a decision cannot be morally good unless it is fair, but it also seems that the only moral issue in such cases is their fairness.

To say that such decisions must be fair is to say that they must be in accord with the Golden Rule, the idea that playing favourites or discriminating against some individuals is without a rational basis and so morally indefensible. In other words, such decisions must be based on an evenhanded application of rational considerations, not simply feelings of preference for some or dislike for others.

The application of this kind of moral consideration to the rationing of health care leads to some unmistakable moral conclusions. For example, as with other social services, it is obviously unfair to limit benefits on the basis of features of potential beneficiaries which are irrelevant to their need for or claim to the benefit. Thus, to deny someone medical treatment because of his or her race or religion is plainly unfair: it would be a clear case of discrimination. Similarly, providing the benefit to one person rather than another because the one is a friend or relative, or in some way 'has connections,' is an obviously unfair form of playing favourites.

The use of age as a basis for limiting entitlements to various social benefits – that is, using the judgment that a person is too old as a ground for denying the benefit – appears generally to be as discriminatory as the use of a person's race or religion. Some people have given this form of discrimination a name: 'ageism.' But in the case of health care entitlement a growing number of people think that denying someone benefits because they are too old is not discriminatory, but justified as an evenhanded application of non-arbitrary and appropriate considerations.

There are a number of arguments for the view that age is a fair basis for rationing health care. Some argue that the just claims of the elderly on at least some kinds of health care resources are very limited, at least in comparison with other groups who need them. This conclusion can be supported by the argument that the elderly have already received their fair share of the benefits of the health care system. This in turn can be supported by an argument like Robert Veatch's according to which the relatively greater opportunity for wellbeing which the elderly have had over the course of their lives weakens their claims on health care in relation to other classes of persons.[2]

But it is not true that all the elderly have made extensive use of the health care system to such a degree that they have exhausted whatever claim they might have on the system. Some people are very healthy throughout their lives and make little or no use of the health care system until their later years. Similarly, many elderly may not have had ample opportunity for wellbeing during their lives, at least in comparison to many other identifiable groups within a society, for example, those with university educations or in higher income brackets. Thus, if the overall extent of one's use of the health care system, or one's overall opportunity for wellbeing are to be taken as just grounds for limiting health care (and it is not at all clear to me that they are just grounds), then it would seem that these features of a person's life, and not his or her age, should be the standard for denying treatment.

Other arguments for the use of a person's age as a basis for limiting health care face a similar problem. For example, one might argue on the basis of purely medical considerations that the elderly are not good candidates for some procedures, such as perhaps, dialysis, organ transplants or bypass surgery. In other words, given the overall condition of the health of elderly patients, such procedures are not likely to be successful. Surely, the overall condition of a person's health is an important factor in determining his or her suitability for some treatments, and equally surely there is some general correlation between a person's age and his or her overall health. But some younger patients are as unpromising as candidates for certain treatments as are the elderly as a group, and some healthy elderly people are as likely to be good candidates for some treatments as anyone else. If the likelihood of benefiting from a treatment is an appropriate condition for providing it when resources are scarce (and it seems to me that condition is morally defensible), then candidates for treatment should be evaluated on the basis of this condition, not age.

Daniel Callahan, who favors the use of age as a basis for rationing health care, accepts this argument of mine. He says:

If we look at a person only as a collection of organs, any given characteristic may well be identical with that found in younger persons (some of whom have wrinkled skin, or failing kidneys, or are bald, or have osteoarthritis, for example). Moreover, even if in some cases, with some conditions, we know age to be generally relevant, we may not know where, on a continuum of characteristics of the aged as a group, any particular old person falls in terms of likely medical outcome. For all these reasons, age as a medical criterion is unreliable.[3]

I believe that this same kind of consideration applies when the issue is not simply whether a given patient is a good candidate medically for some procedure, but concerns the extent of the benefit expected from successful treatment. Suppose that a surgical procedure like bypass surgery or an organ transplant is a scarce medical resource, and that care givers can provide it either to a person who has a life expectancy of five years with the operation or to a person with a life expectancy of ten years with the operation. If there are no other morally relevant considerations, it seems fair to provide the operation to the person with the longer life expectancy. That is the best use of a scarce resource. But, again, the mere fact that one patient is elderly does not by itself settle the issue of life expectancy. There is obviously some correlation between age and life expectancy, but if the latter is the ground for limiting treatment, age becomes strictly irrelevant. That would be so even if age were more tightly correlated with life expectancy than it appears to be.

Considerations about life expectancy are not the only reasons one might have for thinking that a scarce medical resource is better and more efficiently used when given to some rather than others. For example, some treatments enable people having important social obligations to fulfill them, whereas some other people have no similar obligations. But, again, age and social obligation do not correlate perfectly, and, if they did, age itself would not be the decisive factor.

In short, age does correlate with many of the factors which might make it reasonable to deny health care benefits to some people. But it is these factors, not age, which are relevant to fair rationing decisions. Thus, even if there were a perfect correlation between a person's age and one or another of the factors relevant to a fair denial of treatment, it would be these factors, not age, that are morally relevant. But since the correlation is not perfect, the use of age as a sure sign, or even as a strongly presumptive sign, that such a factor is present is unfair. It follows that, if age is to be a fair basis for denying health care benefits, then there must be something about age itself, and not simply things that are correlated with age, which makes limiting entitlements reasonable.

Callahan's book, *Setting Limits*, contains what is probably the best known argument that age itself is a morally acceptable basis for limiting health care. Underlying Callahan's argument is his belief that we have the idea of a 'tolerable death,' that is, a death which, while regrettable in many ways is not premature or untimely, like the death of a young person or even one in middle years. This idea is correlated with the idea of a 'natural life span,' which is not a biological, but a biographical concept. A natural life span is completed when the projects, plans and commitments which constitute a person's life are largely completed, and this usually occurs by a person's late 70s or early 80s.[4]

Callahan believes that when a person has lived out a natural life span, medical care should not be used to resist death, but only to mitigate suffering. His exact argument for these moral judgments is difficult to determine. He is clear, however, that his argument is not that the lives of those who have completed a natural life span lack value. Rather he maintains that this moral judgment 'reflects instead an acceptance of the inevitability of death in general and its acceptability for the individual after a natural life span in particular.'[5]

This hint about the grounds for Callahan's moral judgments suggests that two of the central claims in his book in fact provide the key premises in his argument. The first of these claims is that medicine should have limited aims, in particular, the promotion of the kind of wholeness which constitutes health, and that those aims do not include a relentless effort to resist and stave off death. Resisting death makes sense in the context of seeking to secure for people a complete and satisfying life, and that is achieved when a person has lived out a natural life span.[6]

The second of Callahan's central claims is that there are 'ends of aging,' goals which aging people appropriately pursue. Here Callahan articulates a communitarian vision of human life and value, and argues that the individualistic effort to extend one's life can clash with the more important activities which give meaning to the lives of the aged – such things as giving example and support to the young, revealing the bonds between generations and the continuity of a community over time, and preparing for death.[7]

So perhaps the argument is as follows: the reasonable ends of medicine are limited in such a way that extending lives beyond a natural life span is not part of what the health care system should undertake to do. And this does no harm to the elderly who are denied life extending treatments, since the purposes of their aging are as well or better served by denying them such treatments.

Perhaps the most salient thing about this argument is that it proceeds independently of concerns about the situation created by the scarcity of health care resources. Callahan's book is filled with discussions of costs and the necessity for rationing, and this concern is surely one reason why he is concerned to limit the aims of medicine. But his main argument seems to depend only on his claims about the nature of medicine and of aging. If I read him correctly, Callahan could make his argument even if there were no scarcity of health care resources. This raises suspicions about Callahan's argument as a case for using age as a reasonable basis for rationing, rather than as an argument that extending life beyond a natural life span is not really a good thing to do.

A more fundamental problem with Callahan's argument is an unjustified move from considerations which might motivate some elderly to decline some forms of health care to a conclusion which justifies care givers in denying to the elderly generally health care which many elderly seek, and seek with good reason. Callahan presents considerations which can and often do motivate elderly people in their decisions about whether or not to seek or accept various forms of health care. Some elderly people say and believe that their life is complete, that seeking to extend it is without meaning for them, that such efforts unreasonably interfere with other things they should be doing, and so on. However, many elderly rightly have different evaluations of their lives and future prospects, and are surely justified in seeking life extending health care. The grounds for limiting treatment to which a patient or his or her proxies might appeal in refusing treatments are plainly not sufficient to justify social decisions to deny treatments to classes of people who want them. Moreover, this insufficiency is not overcome by the fact that the class of people to be denied treatment includes many who find particularly compelling the grounds for voluntarily refusing to seek it.

In other words, the central difficulty in Callahan's argument is that factors which make some sense when considered as part of the motivations and interests of some, but not all, elderly people, or of those who have responsibility for making decisions on their behalf, are generalized and objectified so as to ground limits on what society is obliged to provide for just those elderly who have an interest in life extending treatments. This move simply fails to address the question of whether or not this kind of limitation of health care is fair.

Callahan tries to justify this move by appealing to the ideas of the ends of medicine and the ends of aging. But he has given no evidence that there are any such things, over and above the motives and interests of some elderly people and the policy choices and moral constraints which guide the practice of health care. Surely there are certain interests of elderly people, sometimes to be left alone, untreated, (but sometimes to be treated in one or another manner); and surely there are certain forms of help which are more appropriate and some that are less appropriate for the health care system to seek to provide in various circumstances. But these facts about people's interests and about the goals which the health care should be pursuing have no tendency to show that there are such things as the ends of medicine or the ends of aging in the sense Callahan needs for his argument. For he needs ends of aging which justify limiting treatment even when the elderly want it, and ends of medicine which constrain health care providers from giving help they morally and technically can provide.

Furthermore, even if Callahan's generalizations about the ends of aging and of medicine were better grounded than they appear to be, they are simply irrelevant to the issues of fairness which rationing decisions raise. Thus Callahan's argument serves to distract us from facing the difficult questions of fairness we must address squarely when rationing is necessary. If we keep in mind that this is the question we must answer, Callahan's argument loses much of its initial plausibility.

The failure of Callahan's argument, and the other arguments I have touched upon, does not, of course, show that all arguments for using age as a basis for rationing health care are unsound. Indeed, I am aware of one such argument which avoids the specific criticisms I have made against the arguments already considered.[8]

Still, the arguments I have so far presented establish a strong presumption that the use of age as a basis for rationing health care is unfair. For they address most of the intuitions and arguments which underlie the idea that using age as a basis for rationing health care could be fair. This presumption can be strengthened by looking further at some of the factors which can make these intuitions and arguments appealing.

First, it should be noted that the use of age or of any other morally dubious basis for rationing health care is not a necessity. As I have already noted, there are in many of the situations which call for rationing rational grounds for deciding who is to receive and who is to be denied treatment: sometimes there are strictly medical grounds, and sometimes the benefit of treating one person rather than another is obviously greater. Even when such rational grounds are not present, there is a fair basis for deciding: some sort of randomizing procedure such as a lottery.

Second, the distinction between rationing decisions and allocation decisions is important here. For some legitimate allocation decisions can have a negative impact on the health care available to the elderly, and so can appear to be rationing health care on the basis of age. But such decisions are not cases of age discrimination. Rejecting age as a basis for rationing does not imply that, in making allocation decisions, we should give any settled, definite priority to the health needs of the elderly as a group. Thus, if the differences between the moral issues raised by rationing and by allocation decisions are kept in mind, one can address the complexities of allocation decisions which will affect the health care resources available for the elderly without supposing that decisions which limit these resources are decisions to deny them to people just because they are too old.

In other words, if my argument so far is sound, it is wrong to deny any health care service to a person just because he or she is too old. But this does not mean that, in deciding what services to make available and at what levels, we are obliged to provide those services which the elderly especially are likely to need.

Thus, for example, a society could face a choice between either providing basic entry level diagnosis and care that is accessible to all or supporting certain expensive procedures, such as bypass operations or transplants, which are of most utility to elderly patients. In a situation of this kind, it would not be unfair to choose the first alternative, and, indeed, it would seem to be unfair to choose the second. To choose the first would not be age discrimination: no one would be denied a treatment just because he or she is too old, and the unavailability of resources needed to meet these needs of patients, many of whom are elderly, would be a side effect of a decision justly taken for the sake of providing care needed by everyone.

In the real world, allocation decisions are never this simple, but the simple example reveals the moral issue. For it is surely possible that, in a reasonable and completely fair health care system, addressing the common needs of all and the special needs of other disadvantaged groups would so use up the available resources that little would be left to deal with problems which tend to afflict the elderly more than others.

But as I said at the start, allocation decisions differ from rationing decisions in that the former involve more than simple fairness. We can be evenhanded in our help to others and still fail to be just. For we can refuse to provide a level of help which a decent concern for others requires – a level of help we want for ourselves and would give, and feel duty bound to give, to those with whom we identify. When this more complex issue of social responsibility is considered, the health care needs of the elderly, as of other deprived groups, appear to make greater, not lesser demands on our common resources than they now do.[9]

I close with a final point in support of the presumption against using age as a basis for rationing health care. It concerns the negative impact on the elderly, and on social attitudes towards the elderly, which any rationing scheme based on age would have. Norman Levinsky, an American physician, has very powerfully explored these consequences of rationing on the basis of age:

Only if routine medical care were withheld would the savings be substantial. The noneconomic costs of a national policy to restrict routine care for the elderly would be high. To achieve acceptance of such intuitively distasteful measures would require a societal reeducation (brainwashing) effort that would exacerbate tensions between the generations and further devalue the status of the elderly. Restrictions would not, in practice, be applied equitably. A categorical criterion for rationing, such as an age, is appealing to some because it is clear and easy to administer. In my view, the ease of application is a danger, not an advantage. Society must not insulate itself from the agony of each decision to forgo beneficial treatment as it is experienced by patients, families and caregivers. If rationing is only the impersonal application of a rule to a faceless group, we risk an ever-expanding set of exclusions of the elderly from medical care as costs increase.[10]

Notes

1 For a fuller account see my, The right to health care and its limits, in *Scarce Medical Resources and Justice*, Braintree, MA: The Pope John Center (1987), pp. 13–25; my account is a natural law analysis which grounds rights in individual and social obligations. For a general statement of this approach to entitlements, see John Finnis, *Natural Law and Natural Rights*, Oxford: Oxford University Press (1980), pp. 161–228.

2 See Robert Veatch, Justice and the economics of terminal illness, *Hastings Center Report* 18.4 (August/September 1988), 34–40, at 39–40.

3 Daniel Callahan, *Setting Limits: Medical Goals in an Aging Society*, (New York: Simon and Schuster, 1987), p. 166.

4 *Ibid.*, pp. 65–76, 166–71.

5 *Ibid.*, p. 172.

6 *Ibid.*, pp. 61–5.

7 *Ibid.*, pp. 25–51.

8 See Norman Daniels, *Am I My Parents Keeper?* (Oxford: Oxford University Press, 1988), especially pp. 83–102.

9 The remarks in this and the preceding four paragraphs were occasioned by aspects of Daniels, *op. cit.*; although they would be part of a response to Daniels' complex and subtle argument, neither a fair statement of the argument nor a response to it can be developed here.

10 Norman G. Levinsky, Age as a criterion for rationing health care, *New England Journal of Medicine* **322** (1990), 1815.

12

Economic devices and ethical pitfalls: quality of life, the distribution of resources and the needs of the elderly[1]

MICHAEL BANNER

Some while ago I heard a senior administrator give a rather unsatisfactory lecture on the topic of the distribution of resources within the Health Service. It was unsatisfactory not so much because the message of the lecture was that decisions in this area are extremely difficult to take, but because the speaker seemed to think that the repeated insistence on this point would do in lieu of an attempt to state the principles which govern, or at least should govern, the practice.

Decisions about the distribution of resources within the Health Service are important decisions for the obvious reason that the provision of funds for health care does not, and could not, meet all conceivable claims which might be made upon the budget. The Beveridge Report proposed that 'a comprehensive national health service will ensure that for every citizen there is available whatever medical treatment he requires in whatever form he requires it', but no matter how well funded, no health service could be comprehensive in this sense. Governments, civil servants and administrators are obliged, therefore, to allocate resources between the various specialisms, deciding how much is to be devoted to neo-natal care, how much to transplant surgery, how much to the care of the elderly, and so on. These decisions are no doubt extremely difficult, but this is all the more reason to think that we should seek to make them in an informed and principled way. It is not good enough to allow decisions as to the distribution of resources to be generated, so to say, from the interplay of tradition, interests, pressure groups and – what must now be added in the light of the present Government's policies – market forces, for where we allow these decisions to be 'generated' rather than consciously taken, we can hardly be confident that the result will be a morally acceptable, let alone an efficient, use of limited funds.

If it is the case that the distribution of scarce resources has been settled in an unduly *ad hoc* manner, then one must welcome attempts to bring principles to bear on the problem. Unfortunately however, among the various proposals for the rational distribution of resources within the Health Service, the one which is currently most influential ought to cause us considerable concern. For under the guise of bringing properly informed evaluations to the problem of establishing priorities for health care, it threatens to impose extremely questionable moral assumptions on medical practice, and so to undermine medicine's traditional values and its characteristic commitments – such as to the care of the dependent elderly.

The proposal to which I refer has emanated from the Department of Economics at the University of York and is associated with the QALY (Quality Adjusted Life Year) and its inventor, Professor Alan Williams. Now the QALY is intended in the first place as a measure of the good which various health care activities achieve. But in combination with certain other assumptions, and making use of costings of different treatments, it becomes a means by which priorities in the distribution of resources can be settled, and it is clear that Williams and others have promoted the QALY as a solution to this particular problem. Williams writes: 'The essence of a QALY is that it takes a year of healthy life expectancy to be worth 1, but regards a year of unhealthy life expectancy as worth less than 1. Its precise value is lower the worse the quality of life of the unhealthy person (which is what the quality adjusted bit is all about) ... The general idea is that a beneficial health care activity is one that generates a positive amount of QALYs, and that an efficient health care activity is one where the cost-per-QALY is as low as it can be. A high priority health care activity is one where the cost-per-QALY is low, and a low priority activity is one where the cost-per-QALY is high.'[2]

This is a proposal fraught with difficulties, not only moral but also technical or practical. Of the technical or practical problems Williams is not unaware, but of the moral problems he seems largely oblivious. To the practical difficulties I shall only allude, for I shall allege that even if, for the sake of argument, we concede the possibility of solutions to these genuine and deep difficulties, still we ought to conclude, on moral grounds, that Williams' proposal has very little to commend it.

To begin at the beginning it is worth recording the deep misgivings which even the very notion of the 'quality of life' can arouse.[3] It seems to lead us inexorably towards the judgement that some people have a low quality of life, a judgement which is to some reminiscent of the notorious concept of 'life unworthy of life' which was used to justify the abuse of the mentally and physically handicapped, the mentally ill and the elderly under the Nazi regime. To make such judgements, and to conclude as Williams does, that some states of existence register as less than zero on his scale (i.e. as states worse than death) is, it might be felt, the beginning of a slippery slope which may end, for example, in the practice of compulsory euthanasia for those unfortunate enough to be so assessed.

I do not for a moment underestimate the seriousness of the concern thus expressed, but I do think that in fact these worries can be allayed. Of course, the judgement that a particular person has such a low quality of life that death is preferable to further treatment, may be presumptuous and ill-informed and it may even be taken as providing grounds for the killing of patients; were we to look at current practice in relation to the so-called 'care of the newborn', we would almost certainly come across instances of such dubious premises being employed in invalid arguments.[4] But should we reject the very possibility of quality of life judgements just because these might sometimes be misjudgements and, even if not mis-judgements, might sometimes be misused? No doubt we should meet the judgement that such a patient has, in an absolute sense, a low quality of life, with a degree of suspicion. There are aspects of a patient's life which are inherently outside the scope of an observer's scrutiny. It will be replied, however, that we must acknowledge the legitimacy, or at least the necessity, of such judgements in certain circumstances. We shall surely not wish to quibble with the judgement which a sensitive and experienced medical practitioner might reasonably make in declining to pursue heroic measures on behalf of the incompetent patient who, let us say, arrives in an intensive care unit after a major heart attack. And such a judgement seems to be implicitly a quality of life judgement, and one moreover which is absolutely essential to the responsible care of the terminally ill, for example.

We might allow, therefore, that in very particular circumstances the judgement that a patient has a low quality of life, or even such a low quality of life that further measures to preserve life are inappropriate, is one which might be warranted. But we shall add two points. First of all, that to concede this is to concede very little to the case for either voluntary or involuntary euthanasia, which argues not that in such circumstances further measures to preserve life are inappropriate, but rather that in such circumstances measures intended to cause death are permissible. This, however, clearly requires a new argument; it is not, as such, required by the assessment of the situation. The second point would be that even those who feel some unease in presuming to measure the quality of life of a particular patient in particular circumstances, may nonetheless allow the propriety of the comparative judgements on classes of patients which decisions about allocation of resources may require. That is to say, those who hesitate to admit the claim that such and such a patient has a low quality of life, may yet accept the claim that one treatment does more than another (whether alternative treatments for the same complaint, or treatments for different complaints) to enhance the quality of life of a class of patients. And that is all that is required for the use of the concept of quality of life to have a place in the debate over distribution.

If the suspicions I have referred to can, as I think, be allayed, we may happily acknowledge that the concept of 'quality of life' is a useful one, serving to denote an aspect of a patient's well-being which has always been of concern to good medical practice, even if it has only recently been so named. For in acting in the service of health, medicine has always sought to add to a patient's life both quantity and quality, that the patient may not just exist for three score years and ten, but genuinely flourish. Consciousness of quality of life serves to remind the medical practitioner of this fact and is thus an important aid to the profession's thinking. But what of the concept of a QALY? Can this have a similarly benign role?

To see the point of the concept we need to note that though, fortunately, in many cases medicine simply acts in the service of health without having to wonder about the relationship of quality and quantity of life (thus in treating diabetes or in offering kidney dialysis, the doctor will give the patient the chance not only of more life, but of better life), cases are not always that simple. Sometimes a treatment which adds to length of life may so affect the patient's hope of flourishing as to be unacceptable. Thus it may be that radical surgery offers the best chance of remission for a patient with advanced cancer, but a remission so troubled by pain, discomfort or disability as to be a burden and not a benefit. Even in less extreme cases a choice between two forms of treatment may be complicated by the same sort of balance of considerations. An instance which is often cited is concerned with the treatment of laryngeal cancer. The choice for patients with advanced but localised laryngeal cancer is between surgery and radiation therapy. Surgery improves survival at the expense of impaired speech; radiation preserves speech at the expense of a decreased chance of survival.[5] And, to take another example, it may be – though the matter is, of course, controversial – that mastectomy offers the best prospect of long life to a patient with breast cancer, whereas a treatment which avoids such radical surgery is more acceptable on 'quality of life' grounds. The moral is clear and well put by two practitioners: 'we strongly believe that in cancer therapy equal emphasis should be given to the patient's quality of life as well as to objective measurements of tumour progression or regression.'[6]

The patient who has to choose between alternative therapies, or the administrator who has to decide which of two rival approaches to the treatment of the same disease or illness should be funded, will undoubtedly welcome the attempt which is represented by the invention of the QALY to render commensurable the two goods of quantity and quality of life. For the QALY is intended to determine what good a treatment does, weighing both quality and quantity of life together, and so to assist us in the difficult situations which sometimes confront us where quality and quantity conflict. In this respect the QALY may prove to be a useful device.

This said, we are, nonetheless, still a long way from the use of QALYs which Williams intends. However, if the first and most natural use of the concept of quality of life and of the QALY is, as we have said, in considering the merits of alternative courses of treatment open to the individual patient or in pursuit of limited funding, there is surely a temptation to carry it over to cases which are quite different and much more difficult, where the competition is not between alternative therapies for the same treatment but between entirely independent medical specialisms: between, for example, paediatrics and renal surgery, or between terminal care and gynaecology. For if in choosing between alternative therapies for the same treatment, we are naturally sensitive to the contribution each one makes to both quantity and quality of life, should not the administrator be sensitive to the same consideration in choosing between funding independent health care activities? And if so, is not the QALY the very device which will render distribution sensitive in the appropriate way, enabling us to settle the vexed question of priorities in health care? So Williams would contend.

If Williams' proposal for the distribution of resources is to be applicable even in principle – if, in other words, it is genuinely capable of making the comparisons it proposes as essential to rational decision making – then it must, of course, be able to measure both the costs and the benefits of treatment. That is to say, to achieve comparability of alternative health care activities two steps are involved. First of all the proposal requires that we assign different forms of treatment a 'QALY value' – that is, a value which represents the gain to the patient in both quality and quantity of life offered by treatment over against non-treatment. Secondly, it requires that we introduce into our considerations financial assessments of alternative treatments, for it is not just the QALY value – that is the benefit – of a treatment which is of interest to those concerned with the distribution of resources. They will also be concerned with the cost of achieving this QALY value. Thus to take an example of a calculation done by Williams (and cited by Michael Lockwood[7]), a heart transplant is said to have a QALY value of 4·5 and home and hospital dialysis to have QALY values of 6 and 5 respectively. But the costs of these treatments are very different, and once this is taken into account heart transplants represent the best value for money: according to Williams the cost per QALY is £5000 for heart transplants, but £11000 and £14000 respectively for home and hospital dialysis. Thus in comparison with dialysis, heart transplants are in Williams' terms 'a high priority activity'.

In actual fact both of these steps – the measuring of costs and the measuring of benefits – are far from straightforward. Since, however, my final conclusions do not depend on a challenge to the success of these two steps, I shall only pause to note some doubts about the validity and scope of the sort of calculations which Williams' proposal requires, before going on to give attention to the more pressing moral difficulties which beset the policy Williams recommends.

The assessment of the relative priority to be accorded to different health care activities depends first on the calculation of the QALY value of various treatments. Calculation of a QALY value compounds expectations of quality and quantity of life given the treatment in question, over against expectations without treatment. Thus, in an example I have already given, the QALY value of kidney dialysis is the gain to the patient of so many years at such and such a quality above and beyond what can be expected without dialysis – which is, of course, very little indeed. Now one element in the calculation is reasonably amenable to scientific assessment given sufficient research, and that is the increased expectation of quantity of life which various treatments yield. But the second element, the contribution made to quality of life, is by no means as easily assessed. The most commonly used scales of assessment (including the one relied upon by Williams) combine considerations of distress and disability, both of which are important aspects of what we refer to by the concept of 'quality of life'. There are, however, other aspects of it, not included under these heads. And even were it feasible to widen the scope of the benefit to health which is allowed to count, most of us will sense that attempts to assign a value to a person's life under different circumstances are as likely to fall as far short of measuring what we intend by that rich concept 'quality of life' as IQ tests fall short of measuring that wide ranging intellectual ability and commonsense which we describe by the word 'intelligence'.[8]

Nor are the calculations employed to determine the cost of obtaining the QALY benefit easily made or uncontroversial. First of all the notion of 'the cost of treatment' is not a simple one, for, even if one considers only the direct costs of treatment to the Health Service, economists would want to distinguish average cost and marginal cost, fixed costs and running costs.[9] Now depending on which cost you choose as most important you may get very different answers to the question of what a particular activity costs: Drummond and Mooney cite a diagnostic procedure of six sequential tests for detecting colonic cancer which was estimated to cost less than $2500 for each case detected, whereas the marginal cost of carrying out six tests, as opposed to five, was $47 000 000. As they put it, 'clearly it is important to ask the right costing question.'[10] It surely is, but it is by no means clear which is the right question to ask or that the information needed to answer whichever question is the right one is available, for, as Williams points out, there is 'very little routine information on' capital costs.[11] Thus his estimates of the costs of various treatments are usually estimates of marginal costs.

These problems may be soluble. But there is another respect, according to Williams, in which the information on health costs which is readily available is 'not usually suitable as it stands for the efficiency calculus which is our central interest'[12] and this presents a graver difficulty. The limitation on available information is well illustrated by the policy of reducing the length of stay in hospital after treatment. This may or may not represent a saving to the hospital budget, but, as Williams comments, 'the patients' costs are being ignored in all this, as are the costs falling on non-hospital services, local authority social services, voluntary bodies, and friends and relatives who provide support.'[13] Williams is surely right that any calculations of the cost of treatment, no matter how cost is understood, which consider only what we might term the narrowly medical items – the cost of employing the surgeons, of providing a hospital bed, of offering an appropriate regimen of drugs and so on – have a certain unreality about them. There are many other costs associated with treatment or non-treatment, even if not directly charged to the health budget, which seem to have been arbitrarily excluded. To take a current example: the contention that an operation at a hospital 50 miles from the patient's home is cheaper than the cost of the same operation at the local hospital, ignores the considerable cost which relatives may incur in using public transport in order to visit the patient. Or, to take another example, it may be that the average patient seeking a heart transplant is a middle-aged person with a family, and that this family may become a burden on the State if the patient is untreated and remains in poor health or worse. The average patient seeking a hip replacement may be a good deal older and have no such responsibilities, or at least none which are likely to be unfulfilled if he or she goes without treatment. If we are concerned to make a proper estimate of the costs of treatment and non-treatment so as to make a rational use of limited resources ought we not to widen our calculations to consider costs such as these?

So Williams would suggest, it seems. But there are serious reasons to doubt both the feasibility and the desirability of construing 'costs' quite so widely. On the matter of the feasibility of so construing costs, one might think that the calculation of cost becomes meaningful at the expense of being practical when the notion of cost is widened beyond the direct charge on the health budget. But, more importantly, one will surely hesitate to broaden consideration of cost when to do so is to take a step in a direction which very obviously raises the spectre of making provision of health care dependent on social worth.

I pause rather than dwell on the difficulties inherent in calculations of cost and benefit because even if simply as calculations they could be regarded as beyond suspicion, the use which Williams and others make of them is morally questionable. Of course, if we swallowed our doubts about the validity and scope of the measures of benefit and cost, then as calculations they would be unexceptionable and, as I have already acknowledged, of some interest. But Williams requires not only that we accept the validity of his sums, but also the use to which he puts them in proposing that a rational policy for the distribution of resources should aim at producing as many QALYs as possible. That is to say, he proposes that a policy for the distribution of resources should not only be sensitive to considerations of quantity and quality of life, but should be determined by an intention to obtain the maximum number of QALYs our money can buy. He proposes, in words I have already cited, that 'A high priority health care activity is one where the cost-per-QALY is low, and a low priority activity is one where the cost-per-QALY is high.' Thus the QALY becomes a device which measures not just the contribution which various treatments make to quantity and quality of life, but also the relative worth of different health care activities, so that QALY maximisation is, according to Williams, a rational policy for determining the distribution of scarce resources.

Before I criticise that claim it is worthwhile, I think, to consider in broad terms the implications which this 'rational policy' would have for the pattern of provision within the health service. One critic of Williams' proposals (Professor John Harris of the University of Manchester) points out that 'it will usually be more QALY efficient ... to channel resources away from (or deny them altogether to) areas such as geriatric medicine or terminal care'.[14] I think that he is right, and that Williams' 'rational policy' has the same implications for the care of the mentally handicapped, for example; but for the moment I shall consider only geriatric and terminal care.

At first sight it might not seem obvious that a policy of QALY maximisation will accord low priority to the care of the elderly. After all 'Old people need simple things' according to an article on 'Ethical implications in aging' in the *Encyclopedia of Bioethics*, such as decent care for their eyes, teeth and feet.[15] They may, of course, need some basic help to allow them to remain in their homes, but even when they are no longer capable of living on their own they may require only relatively straight-forward, albeit highly skilled and sensitive, nursing. Thus in principle the cost of providing for the care of the elderly is quite low and might be expected to come out reasonably well in a QALY calculation.

The point that we have overlooked, however, is the relatively low expectation of life of the elderly, and the fact that many of the services they need make absolutely no difference to that expectation. Such medical care of the elderly thus provides only an improvement in quality of life and an improvement which will be enjoyed for a much shorter time than if a similar benefit were to have been provided for a younger person. So even where the provision of care for the elderly proves to be relatively cheap, it will yield a small return of QALYs compared with medical activity which either adds length to an otherwise healthy life or adds quality to a life with a long time still to run. This is not to say, of course, that *all* the services from which the elderly benefit will receive unfavourable assessment. According to some of the (inherently questionable) calculations which have been done, hip replacement operations – a procedure often required in early old age – should have a high priority because they render significant benefit at low cost. But it is, I suspect, unusual for the care of the elderly to be so favourably assessed by a policy of QALY maximisation. For the most part, the relatively modest improvements or preservation of quality of life which much of the care of the elderly achieves is likely to be hard pushed to defend itself if asked to compete on these terms.

Professor Harris's point about the low priority QALY calculations will accord to terminal care is also sound. The work of a hospice is aimed not primarily at extending life but at making it more comfortable by palliative care. By the relief of symptoms, particularly by the relief of pain, patients are granted an opportunity to find peace and meaning in their last days, weeks or months, parting from relatives and friends in the best of circumstances. Such work increases a patient's quality of life and some aspects of that increase, such as benefit from the relief of pain, will be registered on the standard scales for measuring quality of life, though no such a scale is likely to be sensitive to the significance or value of dignified human parting. To the extent, then, that the quality of life of the terminally ill is measurable, the hospice can enter into the competition for resources alongside any other health care activity by advertising the QALYs it produces; but insofar as it does not add years to life and adds quality only to those with low life expectancy, it can hardly enter the competition with great confidence of success.

To take seriously a policy of QALY maximisation would result, so it seems, in a considerable devaluing of the care of the elderly and of the terminally ill. Does it follow, then, that our present provision in these areas, often thought in many respects inadequate, is in fact an irrational use of resources which ought properly to be deployed elsewhere in our health service? So we should believe if we accept Williams' contention that a rational policy for the distribution of resources is one which maximises QALYs or health.

It is probably already apparent that Williams' proposal is, broadly speaking, a utilitarian one. It will be apparent too, perhaps, that thus far we have been engaged in the initial skirmishes which always take place with utilitarians, skirmishes aimed at suggesting first of all that the claim to have measured the benefits and burdens which are in question, as is necessary to their calculus, has more than something of pretence about it, and secondly that the policy they recommend is seriously counter-intuitive.

We must, however, do more than skirmish, and unambiguously deny a principle which is central to Williams' proposal. We must contend, in other words, that *the strength of a patient's or class of patients' claim to health care is not, in any straightforward sense, proportionate to the benefit which will be achieved by the treatment of that patient or class of patients, even though it is not irrelevant in certain circumstances to take note of such benefit.* And we make this contention against Williams' policy just because we acknowledge what Williams cannot acknowledge or accommodate, and that is a commitment to justice – to make a point which is standardly made against utilitarians.

What, however, do we mean by 'justice' and what does it demand in this sphere? Were you to browse in a bookshop along a shelf of currently available texts which might provide the answer, your eye might first rest in delight on John Lucas's *On Justice*, with the title's seeming promise of a clear account of the concept. John Rawls' *A Theory of Justice* might cause some anxieties as to the complexity of the problem, and Karen Lebacqz' *Six Theories of Justice* would increase them. But those anxieties would know almost no bounds were you to spot Alastair MacIntyre's *Whose Justice? Which Rationality?*

In fact John Lucas's book does not pretend that the concept of justice is, so to speak, a simple or unitary one. Concerning the principles which should govern distribution of any good, Lucas writes that 'Although ... reasons based on the individual's deeds and agreements are in some way pre-eminent, reasons based on individual need, status, merit, entitlement or right are all, in appropriate circumstances, the proper basis of apportionment. How much weight should be given them will depend partly on the nature of the good, partly on the purposes of the association that has the disposal of the good in question.'[16] And it is MacIntyre's contention, going further than Lucas perhaps, that there are many concepts of justice, each one having its origin in rival social and cultural traditions and only capable of validation by the assessment of the intellectual adequacy of the tradition to which it belongs.[17]

If Lucas and MacIntyre are right, then there is no simple answer to the question which we posed earlier: what is justice and what does it demand in this sphere? Justice will be understood differently and demand different things according to different conceptions of it. And if that is the case, then it is beyond the scope of a paper on the distribution of resources to justify fully the particular conception of justice to which it appeals. All that can be done within such a paper, I suspect, is to elaborate the concept in such a way that those who have an alternative account of justice – or none at all – begin to understand the force of the one which is offered. Fortunately, however, at least one of the concerns which is central to the conception of justice I shall give, is a concern which Williams claims to share, as will emerge in what follows. Thus in criticising his proposals as failing to accord with that conception of justice, I shall be offering a criticism which, by his own standards, he ought to take seriously.

Justice has two major concerns, one to do with fairness and the other to do with need. Neither concern is one which QALY maximisation can cope with, for in making maximisation of benefit the sole ground of distribution this policy cannot countenance the fact that there may be claims to health care which derive strength not merely from the degree of benefit which their satisfaction will realise.

We may speak first of all of fairness, which requires at its most basic level, treating like cases alike, so far as possible.[18] A policy of QALY maximisation, however, since it is concerned only that the good of health be maximised, is inherently insensitive to the question of how that good is allocated between individuals. That is to say, it would prefer a larger benefit for a few over against even only a slightly smaller benefit for many. To take an example: it would prefer to treat nine AIDs patients with slightly better and slightly more expensive drugs and leave one with no treatment (producing remission for each of the nine of 14 months, i.e. a total gain of ten and a half years), to treating all ten with a marginally less good but cheaper alternative supposing that that drug produced a remission of only a year for each patient (i.e. a total gain of ten years). And yet in the face of such a distribution of benefits and burdens the untreated patient would quite reasonably complain that he or she was being treated unjustly. There are some distributions of benefits and burdens which are properly regarded as unjust, no matter that we are assured that the distribution produces the maximum amount of the good which we are concerned to secure. For we should, so far as possible, treat like cases alike. Of course, if we changed the example we have just given, so that the gain from treatment by the slightly more expensive drug is considerably more significant than we have imagined it to be, then it might be right to treat only nine of the ten patients, and indeed we could imagine that this is what the patients themselves would want, provided they had a fair chance to be selected for treatment, by means of a lottery perhaps. But then we should have ensured fairness in another way, bearing further witness to the point that a policy of QALY maximisation, which is intrinsically insensitive to our concern to treat like cases alike, offends against a principle which must be basic to any acceptable distribution of scarce resources.

Fairness is important, and QALYs no doubt offend against it, but a good deal of the debate about the moral implications of Williams' policy for the distribution of resources has been concerned with the question whether QALYs are not only unfair in general but discriminatory in particular against the elderly – whether, that is, they are, as the Americans would say, 'ageist'. This is, I shall suggest, though important, not the main point to make against Williams' proposal. For even were expectation of life excluded from consideration of the problem of distribution, still the claims of the dependent elderly and the terminally ill to treatment would not be properly recognised by Williams just because, given his understanding of need, their need for treatment is small.

It is true, as I have been concerned to argue, that under a policy of QALY maximisation, the elderly will do extremely badly. But one cannot conclude that this in itself is evidence of unfair discrimination and Michael Lockwood thinks that though a policy of QALY maximisation is open to criticism as unjust, the claim made for example by Harris, that the policy would involve such discrimination against the elderly in particular, is unsound.[19]

Lockwood makes the obvious point that there is no improper discrimination involved in preferring some people to others provided the grounds for doing so are relevant to the choice being made. Thus, it is not sexist to prefer strong people for a job which requires physical strength, even if this means that women are not likely to be selected. For women are not rejected because they are women, but because they do not meet a legitimate criterion employed in considering candidates for the job in question. In the same way, a health policy which has a built-in preference for those with a high life expectancy does not discriminate against old people as such. It just so happens that a policy of distribution which is sensitive to life expectancy will tend to favour the young, in the same way that a selection procedure sensitive to physical strength will tend to favour men – though there are in fact some circumstances, according to Lockwood, in which the QALY approach would favour an older over against a younger patient.

As a defence of the QALY policy against this particular objection, however, this answer is, as it stands, inadequate. Preferring people with physical strength does not discriminate against women as such only if the job is of a sort which properly demands physical strength. If the same criterion were used in selecting candidates for, let us say, an academic position, then it would be judged to be discriminatory. It thus begs the question in favour of the QALY policy to say that it is not discriminatory as such when just what is in dispute is whether or not a policy for the distribution of resources for health care ought to be sensitive to life expectancy. The question is whether in preferring those with a higher life expectancy (and thus, in most cases, the young), the QALY approach employs a criterion which is patently appropriate to the distribution of resources. Nor is it to the point in rebutting the charge of discrimination merely to note that there are some circumstances in which it so happens that the policy might actually favour the elderly: such as in choosing between the treatment of a young person with a terminal disease from which he or she will shortly die and the treatment of an older person who has a life expectancy of another ten or so years. It would hardly serve to show the non-discriminatory nature of a policy for the selection of police officers favouring those with four grandparents born in Britain to point out that it did not pick out ethnic minorities as such, and that in some peculiar cases it might actually help them.

The charge that a policy of distribution on the basis of QALY maximisation is discriminatory can only be answered by an argument which shows that life expectancy or age is a factor to which such distribution ought to be sensitive. And it would need to be an argument sufficient to deal with a counter-argument which appeals to our indebtedness to the elderly for their past contributions to society, thus claiming for them a privileged entitlement to proper health care. Now there is such an argument which is widely canvassed and which Harris and Lockwood call the 'fair innings argument'. If it works, it would, according to the latter, not only justify a policy of preferring the young to the old but also show that a policy of QALY maximisation is, if anything, insufficiently 'discriminatory' in relation to the elderly. This argument says that the fact that the elderly have already had a 'decent innings' provides a reason for giving scarce resources to the young who have yet to enjoy a comparable spell (though it is usually not specified how many years constitutes a decent innings). The suggestion is that it would be unfair to treat someone who has enjoyed a full life in preference to one who has not. Thus even if a policy of QALY maximisation happened to favour an older patient in very particular circumstances, this argument, based so it seems on considerations of fairness, insists that the younger patient be preferred.

Whilst there is something in this argument, it needs some fairly careful qualification. Harris is probably right in his contention that 'We should remember that the fair innings argument is only plausible in extreme emergency when hard choices have to be made.'[20] One such emergency might arise where a choice has to be made between two victims of an accident both of whom arrive at an intensive care unit which has space and equipment for only one more patient. Here it *might* be right to choose a young patient for treatment, over against an elderly patient, where both will die without it, so that there may be circumstances in which we would reckon there to be no unfairness in taking age or life expectancy as a relevant factor in making some medical choices. But it is one thing to recognise such a point, and quite another to concede the whole case to those who hold, as in effect advocates of a policy of QALY maximisation do, that in all circumstances claims to medical care are dependent, in some degree, on life expectancy. Certainly Williams' proposal could not be warranted merely by the consideration of hard cases of the sort just mentioned, for outside these extreme situations it would almost certainly be thought unfair to consider differences of say, a year or two in life expectancy as a relevant factor in determining entitlement to treatment.

A policy of QALY maximisation would be unfair in a variety of ways, and unfair in particular to the elderly. But then it might be replied that in all sorts of ways the present pattern of distribution of resources is itself manifestly unfair, and does not treat like cases alike. Some twenty years ago, in 1971, Dr Julian Tudor Hart wrote an article in *The Lancet* in which he argued that the situation was even worse than that, and he formulated what he termed 'the inverse care law', which held that 'the availability of good medical care tends to vary inversely with the need of the population served.'[21] Nearly ten years later in April of 1980, the then Secretary of State for Social Services, Patrick Jenkin, received the Report of the Working Group on Inequalities in Health, subsequently known, after its Chairman, as the Black Report. In considerably greater detail than Hart provided, the Report demonstrated the deep social inequalities in the provision of health services within Britain – and demonstrated it so clearly that the Secretary of State, rather than have the Report properly printed and distributed by his department, made available only some 260 duplicated copies during the August bank holiday week of the year in question when the Establishment was in deepest recess; a tactic which came to nothing however, since it was quickly perceived that a Report which the Government so clearly reckoned to be dangerous must be worth reading, resulting in considerable publicity for it and its eventual publication as a Pelican book.[22]

Since the present distribution of resources for health care is inequitable, criticism of Williams' proposal should not be taken as a justification of the *status quo*. But against Williams' proposal it must be recorded that it would produce unfairnesses of its own – albeit probably not unfairnesses which would correlate as closely with social class as do the present ones – and so cannot be regarded as a satisfactory solution to the problem we are trying to address.

Justice, so I have said, is not just a matter of fairness. It has another aspect, and that is the recognition of need. To distribute goods fairly is to distribute to like cases in like degree, but need in turn justifies – makes just – a distribution which is not an equal split between all the parties who would benefit, but which takes note of the fact that some of those who would benefit have greater need than others, to health care or whatever else is in question.[23] It may be, for example, that a certain patient would benefit in a variety of ways from a kidney transplant, even though kidney dialysis, which he or she presently receives, will ensure moderately good health for the foreseeable future. But certainly this patient, even if he or she could be said to need a kidney transplant, could not be said to need it in quite the same way that someone needs a liver transplant, without which they will be dead in a matter of days. And the greater the need, the greater the claim on resources.

Can a policy of QALY maximisation make any sense of the obligation that just distribution should recognise need? Williams seems to think that it can, and in a discussion of the recent proposals for the reform of the Health Service he defends what he terms an 'egalitarian perspective' which holds that the objective of the Health Service is to meet needs, and to do so as efficiently as possible. What however, is meant by need? He comments that 'Need is a slippery concept which I am going to take to mean "capacity to benefit" for I cannot see how anyone can really "need" anything that will not do them any good. Doing good in health care means increasing people's life expectancy and/or improving their quality of life by reducing health-related disability and distress. So improving the efficiency of the NHS means generating as much of these benefits as possible, given the resources (human, material, and financial) that are available.'[24]

The confusions in this statement ought to be manifest. Whilst it might be true that no one has a need for treatment which will do them no good, so that to have a need for treatment one must have a capacity to benefit from it, it does not follow that everyone who has a capacity to benefit from health care has a need for it. If I am sufficiently vain I may benefit from cosmetic surgery to improve the shape of my perfectly normal, if not perfect, nose, but it is by no means obvious that I have a need for such surgery. Furthermore, and more importantly, it is not the case that need is proportional to capacity to benefit, as Williams seems to think in proposing that a commitment to meeting need entails the maximising of benefit. Were need proportional to capacity to benefit, then the policy of QALY maximisation which puts the claims of the terminally ill or the dependent elderly near the very bottom of the pile could not be faulted on these grounds, just because few benefits accrue to patients treated in these circumstances. Since, however, the need of the terminally ill patient for palliative care is quite clearly greater than the 'need' of the patient for cosmetic surgery, or the need of the patient we imagined as wanting a kidney transplant (no matter that the QALY calculation would probably be in favour of the last two over the first), we can see that Williams offers not a recipe for meeting need, but a device which systematically fails to recognise it.

The question must be asked, however, whether the recognition of need can be built into a feasible policy for the distribution of resources. In the first place we can imagine the point being put that all those who would benefit from health care in fact need it, give or take certain contentious claimants, such as those seeking cosmetic surgery, for example. So, far from providing grounds for discrimination, consideration of patients' needs merely intensifies the dilemma involved in distributing scarce resources. Is there any way, then, in which we can distinguish between the claimants for health care as more or less in need?

Need does seem to admit of degrees, though not in the way Williams supposes, for there are certain sorts of needs which stand out from the crowd of general and lesser needs as making a particular claim upon us. They are, for example, the needs of those whose lives are endangered by illness or injury, the needs of the dependent elderly, the needs of the seriously handicapped, and the needs of the terminally ill.

Now the claim which some of these needs make on health care is a claim which the advocate of QALY maximisation might pretend to explain. If you think of need as capacity to benefit, then the need of someone with acute appendicitis is one which will be recognised just because the treatment of such a patient will show up well in QALY calculations. But in this way of thought, the other needs I have mentioned will receive no special recognition. Indeed the needs of the terminally ill, the dependent elderly, and of the mentally and physically handicapped will be, as I have said, low priority needs, for the meeting of them will inevitably represent a poor return in QALY terms.

The misunderstanding of need which a policy of QALY maximisation involves, might have been avoided had attention been given to the simple fact that though care of the dependent elderly, of the terminally ill, or of the mentally and physically handicapped, produces a 'poor return', this does not undermine the commitment of those engaged in the giving of such care. The nurse who devotes a year of patience and sympathy of quite heroic proportions to enabling a single stroke patient to achieve some modest goal such as being able to button a shirt, does not do so because he or she has made the mistake of supposing that perhaps far greater things were possible which might have rendered the endeavour worthwhile if they had been achieved. Indeed the devotion to such care is surely founded on the insight that the slight amelioration which these conditions admit of, far from being a reason for thinking care so directed to be problematic, dubious or marginal, as the QALY maximiser must suppose, is instead the explanation of the peculiar and particular strength of the claim which it makes upon us and our resources. This might, at first sight seem paradoxical, but it is not really so. The point is that in these particular circumstances, where we can do very little, we have a special obligation to do what we can.

The question which the advocate of QALY maximisation will ask, namely 'why should we invest so much in what promises so little return?', is one which evidences a failure to recognise the demand made upon us by the existence of those whose needs are so patent partly because human endeavour can do so little to meet them. Thus we should see in the attempt to meet those needs as best we can, not an inefficient or unproductive use of resources, but rather something which is at the heart of humane medicine as it is at the heart of a humane, or we might just say human, society: that is, the expression of a sympathy which asserts a desire to maintain, and does indeed maintain, our kinship and community with those who, through the approach of death or through physical or mental deprivation, stand in different ways on the edges of the most limited and perhaps the most obvious of communities, namely the community of those who are fit, strong and productive.[25]

Paul Ramsey has written that 'to comprehend the depth and scope' of the Biblical notion of justice, 'it is necessary first to *distinguish* ... two kinds of justice – God's judgemental righteousness and human justice – and then to *relate* them decisively together, so that the meaning of God's righteousness acting in judgement ... becomes normative for human justice.'[26] Were we to allow ourselves to speak now in a theological voice we would refer to this work amongst the elderly and the handicapped as expressive of a fidelity towards them in which we rightly see a reflection of the trustworthy fidelity of God himself towards human kind; fidelity to the elderly on our part, so understood, is an attempt to allow our justice to approach, as its required pattern, the justice of God. We would say, further, that the commitment of some to the care of the elderly and the handicapped is a response to a divine vocation to reflect in this sphere of human life the continuing and unbroken fidelity of God, just as the vocation to marriage, for example, seeks to express it in another. So that we shall find ourselves insisting that this work is to be valued not only in and of itself, but also because the expression of solidarity and fidelity which it involves is a sign or reflection of, and thus a faithful response to, the gracious work of God in keeping faith or community with us in Jesus Christ.

To return from where it would have been better, in other circumstances, to have begun, we may repeat the claim that in considering need, justice has an eye for the most needy. In traditional portrayals, the figure of justice wears a blindfold. The blindfold symbolises justice's impartiality, an impartiality which suggests that justice treats all who make claims upon her equally. And this, in part, is right as I have wanted to say in speaking of justice as fairness. But justice, properly speaking, peaks under the blindfold and sees cases of need. And in particular justice is partial to the very needy and gives a priority to their claims upon her, so that we can indeed say that the claims which, for example, the dependent elderly, the handicapped and the terminally ill make upon us are primary amongst the claims of all those in need.

Is it possible to be more exact, however? Can the claims of need and of the very needy be ranked, so that our administrators are given a clearer guide in setting priorities? Perhaps there is more to say than I am capable of saying, but I doubt that even at the end of discussions more insightful than these, a graph or a table could be produced which would take us beyond what has thus far been said, namely that we cannot regard the claims of those in need, and in especial need, as merely some claims among the claims of all those to whom we might do good.

But then the question comes back all the stronger. Can the administrator who must allocate scarce resources accommodate considerations of this sort? Are we not still a long way from offering a workable account of the principles which should govern the distribution of resources? Our discussion suggests that, though we should in principle do the most good we can, we must also bear in mind an obligation to treat like cases alike, and recognise the claims of need. But to this, the proponents of QALY maximisation can be expected to protest that they are looking for something altogether sharper, and indeed we find Williams complaining of opposition to his proposals that 'There is no shortage of rhetoric about "equality" and "need", but most of it is vacuous, by which I mean it does not lead to any clear operational guidelines about who should get priority and at whose expense.'[27]

Now I have not denied that we need to provide a proper answer to the question 'who should get priority and at whose expense?', and I have agreed that we cannot rest content with the present pattern of distribution of health care. Nor am I unaware of the increasing strains which will be placed on the health budget by, for example, the sharp rise which is expected over the next fifty years in the proportion of the population over the age of seventy. The question will thus become the more pressing. Even so I would insist that Professor Williams' protest against his critics gets things the wrong way round. Reflection on the problem of the distribution of scarce resources has to begin by considering what values or principles must be respected in any scheme which could commend itself as morally acceptable. Then we shall have to go on to think about the different problem of how we could give effect to these principles and values in practice, in itself a very serious and important task. It is, nonetheless a secondary task, so that it is to turn the matter on its head to suppose that we should allow the demand for clear operational guidelines to determine what values can or cannot be allowed to enter into our deliberations. The desire for administrative clarity is a legitimate one, but such clarity ought not to be achieved by discounting values, such as justice, which make the task of devising guidelines more difficult. We are under no obligation to prune our values in deference to a desire to make our moral lives more susceptible of 'rational' arrangements. Indeed the obligation is the other way round. It is not that our values must be set aside if they prove recalcitrant in the hands of tidy-minded administrators, but rather that a 'rational' distribution of resources has no claim on our attentions unless it expresses our values, unless it has struggled, for example, to relate the claim that health care should be efficient to the claims of those in need, rather than solved the difficulty by ignoring an element of the dilemma.

A further point must be made, however, and that is that one detects in Williams' discussions of this problem not so much a reasonable demand for 'clear operational guidelines' as an unreasonable demand for an algorithm. Of course, administrators must have clear guidelines which allow them to ensure that their decisions respect whatever principles are regarded as central to a sound policy for the distribution of resources. They cannot be expected to act according to such principles if, for example, the principles are hopelessly unclear or contradictory. But if those principles are not at fault in this respect, it does not follow that administrators lack clear guidelines just because the stated principles do not suggest the sort of simple algorithm which Williams offers with his proposal to maximise QALYs. Williams is foisting on us a very particular paradigm of what it is to offer guidelines, and one which in all sorts of areas of life we reject. To take just one example, judges presented with a statute which forbids unreasonable noise would not complain that, unless they are given an instruction which relieves them of the need for judgment – such as 'all noise over ten decibels is unreasonable' – then they lack clear guidelines. In the same way, administrators who are asked to distribute resources with an eye on fairness and need, as well as on benefit, have no necessary ground of complaint just because they are being asked to exercise a certain amount of judgment rather than merely to do sums.

In answer then, to Williams' complaint, I would claim that these discussions have provided at least the outline of a policy for the distribution of resources and that we have said rather more than the anecdotal administrator with whom we began. 'It is very difficult' is not the basis for a policy, and I have tried, in pointing to the claims of justice which require that we treat like cases alike and give prior claim in health care to cases of need, to offer an account of some of the constraints which a policy for the distribution of resources must acknowledge if it is to be more acceptable than Professor Williams' unsatisfactory proposals. Of course I have not tried to work out the implications of this policy in detail, nor do I suggest that it would be easy to do so. But it may just be that there are no easy solutions, of the sort some economists might like, to the vexed problem of the distribution of resources. Whether or not that is the case, we should certainly not allow a desire for administrative simplicity to override the claims of fairness and need which any policy for the distribution of limited resources must respect if it is to commend itself to our moral reason. Instead we should require that such a policy endeavour to reflect the values which are characteristically expressed in the practice of medicine, including the values which are expressed in the care of the elderly.

Notes

1 I am grateful to Dr Charles Elliott, Mr Luke Gormally, Professor John Harris, Professor Oliver O'Donovan and Dr Nicholas Sagovsky for their criticisms of a draft of this paper and to Professor Basil Mitchell, Dr Michael Lockwood, Dr Solomis Solomou and Dr Jane Wheare for discussions of the topic.
2 The value of QALYs, *Health and Social Service Journal*, July 1985, 3.
3 This was the experience of a Working Party at the Ian Ramsey Centre, Oxford, whose discussions are now published by the Centre as *Quality of Life and the Practice of Medicine*.
4 For some examples see certain cases discussed by R. Weir, *Selective Nontreatment of the Handicapped Newborn*, New York, 1984.
5 B. J. McNeil, R. Weichselbaum and S. G. Parker. Speech and survival: trade-offs between quality and quantity of life in laryngial cancer, *The New England Journal of Medicine*, 1981, 982–7.
6 See T. J. Priestman and M. Baum. Evaluation of quality of life in patients receiving treatment for advanced breast cancer, *The Lancet*, April 24, 1976, 899–901.

7 Michael Lockwood. Quality of life and resource allocation, in *Philosophy and Medical Welfare*, ed. J. M. Bell and S. Mendus (Cambridge, 1988).

8 John Broome makes the further point that 'It is a weakness of QALYs as a measure of good that they ignore many aspects of good', that is to say that they are narrowly focussed on health considerations, whereas the value of a year of good health to one person may be greater than to another, just because of other circumstances, such as their material conditions; 'Goodness, fairness and QALYs', in *Philosophy and Medical Welfare*, ed. Bell and Mendus, 66.

9 See P. Wiles, *Price, Cost and Output*, 2nd. ed. (Oxford, 1961).

10 M. Drummond and G. Mooney, *Essentials of Health Economics* (Aberdeen, 1983), 4.

11 A. Williams. Efficient management of resources, in the National Health Service, in H. S. E. Gavelle and A. Williams, *Health Service Finance and Resource Management* (London, 1980), 68.

12 A. Williams, *ibid*, 67.

13 A. Williams. The Budget as a (mis-) information system, in *Economic Aspects of Health*, ed. A. J. Culyer and K. G. Wright (London, 1978), 88.

14 J. Harris. More and better justice, in *Philosophy and Medical Welfare*, ed. Bell and Mendus, 80.

15 D. Christiansen. Ethical implications in aging, in *Encyclopedia of Bioethics*, ed. W. T. Reich (New York, 1978).

16 J. Lucas. *On Justice* (Oxford, 1980), 164–5.

17 A. MacIntyre. *Whose Justice? Which Rationality?* (London, 1988).

18 The most thorough critique of a policy of QALY maximisation as unfair is to be found in John Harris's 'EQALYty', in *Health, Rights and Resources: King's College Studies 1987–8*, ed. P. Byrne (London, 1988) and the reader is referred to that article for a fuller treatment of this question.

19 Lockwood. Quality of life and resource allocation (see[7]).

20 Harris. EQALYty, 119 (see[18]).

21 J. T. Hart. The inverse care law, *The Lancet*, 1971, i, 405–12.

22 *Inequalities in Health: The Black Report*, ed. P. Townsend and N. Davidson (Harmondsworth, 1982). See also J. Le Grand. The distribution of public expenditure: the case of health care, *Economica*, 1978 (45), 125–42.

23 This is a key point in Michael Lockwood's criticism of QALYs in his paper 'Quality of life and resource allocation', and I have drawn extensively on his argument in what follows. I am inclined to the view, however, that he does not stress sufficiently the problem which respect for the claims of need creates for this particular approach to the allocation of resources.

24 A. Williams. Creating a health care market: ideology, efficiency, ethics and clinical freedom; Occasional Papers of the Department of Economics, York, 1989, 8. A. J. Culyer offers an essentially similar definition and seems to draw the same implication from it, namely that 'the health services exist to minimise need or, what is the same thing, to effect the maximum increase in the health status of the client population'; see A. J. Culyer. Needs, values and health status management, in Culyer and Wright, *Economic Aspects of Health*, 10. Drummond and Mooney seem to endorse this approach to the understanding of need. Need, they say, cannot be determined 'objectively'. 'It is a relative, dynamic, value-laden concept. "Need", as Cooper remarked, "is in the eye of the beholder". Some needs will yield large benefits if met, some will be expensive to meet. Need should be met in different ways and to different extents and weighed up in terms of the costs and benefits of

different courses of action.' See Drummond and Mooney, *Essentials of Health Economics*, 18. And Professor Williams' colleague, Professor Alan Maynard, also regards 'the allocation of health care resources on the basis of need or maximising improvements in health status (QALYs)' not as alternative policies, but as different descriptions of the same policy. See his 'Markets and health care', in *Health and Economics*, ed. A. Williams (London, 1987), 196.

25 Just as the supposition that the rationale of trying to meet the needs of the most needy lies in the prospects of success, conceals from view the true nature of the values which medicine, perhaps unknown to itself, expresses in the care of the dependent elderly and the mentally and physically handicapped, so too does the attempt to portray the case for proper provision for the old as a matter of prudence, since we shall all, one day, be old. For an example of such a strategy, see N. Daniel's *Am I My Parents' Keeper: An Essay on Justice Between the Young and the Old* (Oxford, 1988).

26 P. Ramsey. *Basic Christian Ethics* (Chicago, 1950), 4.

27 A. Williams. Ethics and efficiency in the provision of health care, in *Philosophy and Medical Welfare*, ed. Bell and Mendus, 111.

13

The Aged: non-persons, human dignity and justice

LUKE GORMALLY

There are many kinds of argument about the allocation of resources in the field of health care and there are many different contexts in which such arguments are pursued. There are arguments around the Cabinet table, at regional health authority level, at district health authority level; these arguments issue in the decisions which effectively allocate resources.

Other participants in debate, such as academics of a variety of kinds, argue about the effective arguments. Health care economists, health policy analysts, political scientists, and even philosophers critically evaluate the lines of reasoning of the decision makers. Sometimes the meta-arguments (the arguments *about* the decision makers arguments) begin to influence the decision makers. They change the terms of reference and the concepts that the decision makers use. The most influential academics in this respect are probably the health care economists. Over the last 25 years economic decline in Britain has shifted thinking about the National Health Service (NHS) from a focus on inputs to a focus on outputs. There was a time when improving the NHS was discussed primarily in terms of improving inputs, that is, putting more resources into it. Now that resources are in real terms almost static the emphasis is on outputs – on getting the best value for the limited resources available. It is in this context that health care economists have been influential in developing measures of output, of which the most controversial is the QALY, which was the subject of the previous chapter by Michael Banner. The QALY purports to represent the worth of a treatment, or of a health care intervention, by a mathematical value representing the extra life secured by the intervention, modified by a measure of the quality of that life. Michael Banner has shown in the previous chapter how a policy of QALY maximization would systematically marginalize the elderly in relation to health care provision.

QALYs are not the subject of this chapter and are referred to here simply to illustrate the way academic, second-order argument can influence the first-order argument which yields the decisions about resource allocation. Second-order argument alters first-order argument by changing the terms of the argument, introducing new ways of thinking and an altered sense, therefore, of the possible options.

In this chapter I want to discuss *one* way in which certain practitioners of another academic discipline – philosophy – may reframe the question of what it is to be just in the allocation of resources for medical care of the dependent elderly. Philosophers tend to influence first-order practical thinking on a much longer time-scale than economists. But in a society which is deeply divided over moral issues, such as justice, there is plenty of scope for the influence of philosophical thinking. Philosophy is sometimes a source of wisdom, as it purports to be; but more often it is a source of rationalizations for the bad choices people are inclined to make.

The earlier part of David Hunter's chapter makes clear the demographic background against which the debate about health care of the elderly is occurring. The overall picture is clear: an increasing volume and percentage of dependency among the very old. Against this background people are exercised by the question of what is owed to the elderly in the provision of health care. In offering answers to this question they may rely on differing assumptions. Some of the crucial assumptions concern:

who the elderly are to whom health care is owed;

what is to be included under the notion of health care provision;

who it is who owes the provision of health care to the elderly.

In this chapter I hope to illuminate the way an influential current in contemporary philosophy is tending to revise our common understanding of the first type of assumption – about who the elderly are to whom health care is owed.

We need to take stock of two related lines of thought which would lead to restricting health care entitlement among the elderly to a defined sub-group of that part of the population. The lines of thought in question have already been influential in the answers proposed to a number of other questions about what is morally decent in the practice of medicine. May one carry out destructive non-therapeutic experimentation on human embryos? May one intentionally kill unborn babies? May one kill handicapped newborn babies? Affirmative answers have been given to all three of these questions. One influential line of thought which yields such a response rests on an explanation of what is required if a human life is to have value. Another line of thought yielding the same response rests on an account of what is required for a human being to have basic human rights.

The value of human life

There is widespread scepticism in our society about the existence of a range of basic values which would supply an essential part of the foundation for an agreed understanding of human well-being. If there are no objective values then what account is one to give of the value of individual human lives? An influential answer to this question runs roughly as follows: your life has value in so far as you are in a position to value things and you regard things as valuable. This means that if you do not possess the mental equipment which makes it possible for things to seem valuable to you then there is no account one can give of the inherent value of your life. Human beings who do not possess the mental wherewithal to make things matter *to them* do not *in themselves* matter.

On this account a human being can *give* worth and dignity to his life in so far as he is able to maintain a sense of things and projects being worthwhile and valuable. The corallary to this account of the value of a human life is that those lacking the mental equipment to confer value on their own lives must depend on others to attach value to their lives. This means in practice that if those one would normally expect to value the life of an unborn child or a newborn child (the child's parents) or the life of a senile parent (his or her children) do not themselves reckon that life valuable, then not only is there unlikely to be a social basis for treating that life as valuable, but there is no account to be given of its value.

The basis of human rights

A number of philosophers influential in debates about the ethics of abortion, care of the handicapped newborn and euthanasia, have argued that only a subclass of human beings, namely (as they would say) 'human persons', possess a 'serious right to life' (in the sense of a right not to be murdered.). Their reasoning to this conclusion has gone roughly as follows. In order to possess a right – *any* right – you must have a desire for whatever it is that the right is a right *to*. But in order to have a desire you must possess the concepts which are employed in articulating the desire. This is held to mean that the necessary conditions for possessing a right to life are (a) that you possess a concept of yourself as a perduring entity, and (b) you want to perdure precisely as that entity. Views differ about the stage in childhood development at which one would expect someone to have acquired the concept of himself as a perduring entity. Clearly people also lose the ability to perceive themselves in this way.

The upshot of both lines of reasoning – about the value of a human life and about human rights – is that a distinction is to be drawn between human beings who cannot be said to be 'persons' and those who can be described as 'persons' precisely because they possess *presently exercisable* abilities for reflection, choice and communication.

On one account only persons, in the defined sense, can be thought of as possessing value in their own right, though the value derives from finding things and projects valuable which others may consider there is no reason to think valuable. On the other account, only persons, in the defined sense, possess human rights.

The practical conclusion to be drawn from both accounts is that while there may be intrinsic objections to killing 'persons' there are no intrinsic objections to killing human beings who are not 'persons' (in this special sense of the term 'person'). There may be *extrinsic* objections, such as that a human being is valued by some person, or that the death of a human being would frustrate satisfaction of the desires of some person. The value of partially developed, or defective, or senile human beings becomes, then, a function of the desires of those in a position to value them.

If old people with advanced demetia have not got a right not to be murdered, *a fortiori* they surely are not owed the provision of health care. When we have a large population of old people over the age of 85, 45% of them highly dependent, 20% of them with senile dementia, it will be hard to resist the attractions of the thought that not only do we not owe health care to the demented, but that we can solve our problem at a stroke by eliminating them.[1] It is certain that if we fail to provide satisfactory care for these old people the temptation to kill them will become very strong.

It is important not to underestimate the influence of the argument about 'personhood'; it has shown how serviceable it is in rationalizing the practices of non-therapeutic embryo experimentation, of abortion, and of neo-natal euthanasia. The argument would certainly reach to rationalizing senicide, in the sense of the intentional killing of the senile elderly.

The alleged dependence of rights on special 'personhoood' status quite generally entails a radical restriction of the domain of justice to those with presently exercisable capacities for reflection, choice and communication. In regard to resource allocation, significant numbers of the dependent elderly would be extruded from the domain of distributive justice.

Resisting the revision

The above is intended to illuminate the way an influentiual tendency in contemporary philosophy would revise our common assumption about who the elderly are to whom health care is owed. Our common assumption is that it is owed to *all* the elderly. The revised assumption would be that it is owed to those only among the elderly who are not demented or seriously retarded. The revision should be vigorously resisted, since if it succeeds our society would fail radically by those requirements of justice which should be respected in *any* social arrangement. Why?

First, because justice, in the sense of respect for basic human rights, relies on the assumption that all human beings, *simply in virtue of their humanity*, possess inherent worth. Possession of basic rights is entailed by possession of that inherent worth or dignity. The view that you require something over and above our common humanity in order to possess basic human rights is a view which underpins various forms of exploitation. Opposition to such exploitation tends to rely on a doctrine of human equality, but this doctrine has a sure foundation only if we can see value in the one respect in which human beings are indeed equal – that they are all living members of the human race.[2] If humanity itself has no value, then to say all men are equal is empty rhetoric. The point to saying they are equal is to explain why it cannot be a matter of choice whom we shall treat justly and whom we shall not treat justly.

Bernard Williams has lucidly explained how the attempt to connect basic human rights (like the right not to be murdered) with the possession of 'personhood' (in the sense explained earlier) is a recipe not for justice but for the arbitrariness characteristic of injustice. He has pointed out that almost all the characteristics in terms of which certain philosophers explain the idea of a person 'such as the capacities for responsible action, for relations with others, for first personal reflection, and so on, come in degrees. Moreover, they come in different degrees, and are not simply correlated with each other, nor with different ages, states of mental health or other attributes.' So the idea of a person as these philosophers use it 'will provide no firm basis for rules about killing and similar matters, and those who place faith in it are deceiving themselves. What degree of what characteristics will count in a given context for being a person may very well turn out to be a function of the interests involved – *other people's interests in many cases*. Certainly there is no slippery slope more perilous than that extended by a concept which is falsely supposed not to be slippery.' (Williams 1985, 137; emphasis added)

Implications for public policy

Respect for the dignity of the incompetent elderly is threatened in our society. There are already too many people who intellectually are on a slippery slope that would dispose them to solve the problem of care for the dependent elderly by eliminating the seriously demented. To do that would not only gravely wrong those killed, and corrupt those who did the killing, but would further seriously undermine that respect for the dignity of every human being which is fundamental to the life of any community worthy of the allegiance of decent citizens. We need to resist any tendency in that direction, and for that reason we need as a society to guarantee good quality continuing care for all the elderly who require it.

A second reason for such a social commitment arises from consideration of the other basic value which is threatened by restricting entitlement to health care resources to the non-demented elderly: the value of solidarity with those elderly who are frail and vulnerable.

In relation to those from whom they might expect support, the elderly are parents or belong to a parental generation. To abandon them involves a refusal to recognise a basic indebtedness which is of the essence of our humanity: it is *through* our parents that we come to exist at all. Human beings at the beginning and end of their lives are dependent and vulnerable. Acceptance and care of the elderly in this dependence and vulnerability are not merely owing to them, but need to be shown by a younger generation if it is realistically to recognise the nature of our humanity. It would be disastrous for any human community systematically to abandon care of the elderly weak and vulnerable *because of their weakness*. But that would occur in a distributive scheme from which certain of the debilitated elderly were excluded precisely because of their debility.

Conclusion

The threats to justice and human solidarity represented by the influential philosophical tendency examined in this chapter should not be discounted. They should not be discounted because that philosophical tendency has shown itself to be very amenable to rationalizing bad choices. And the temptations to bad choices in relation to providing proper health care for the debilitated elderly arise from a variety of factors: the increasing demand for such care, the demand in the NHS to improve 'output' from investment, the absence of clear policy commitments, and the general tendency in our culture to prefer convenience to justice.

Precisely because of the temptations, together with the rationalizing tendency, it seems clear that the elderly requiring long-term care have *special* claims on the allocation of resources. For we need as a society to demonstrate an unambiguous commitment to the dignity of the dependent aged and our solidarity with them. The commitment needs to be clear and unambiguous in an age in which influential voices are advocating in effect the abandonment of these values.

In broad terms what is *minimally* required in the provision of health care for the debilitated elderly is a quality of care which so far as possible reduces the temptation to doctors, nurses and others to think that they would do better to kill some of their patients rather than provide them with manifestly inadequate care, in other words care of a kind which leads to rapid deterioration or which fails to palliate. The inadequate care of patients creates the temptation to dispose of patients who are obviously held in low esteem. By contrast, adequate care signifies that the patients are valued.

Notes

1 In Britain there is a tendency, when discussing the desirability of ridding ourselves of the dependent and debilitated, to emphasise the relief this will bring to families. The geriatrician Mary Bliss exemplifies this when she argues that it would ease the economic and other difficulties of families burdened by the care of elderly and incompetent parents if their children were entitled to decide to have their parents killed (Bliss 1990). But there is a potentially larger social agenda than relief of families behind the drive to non-voluntary euthanasia, anticipated in a recent letter to *The Times* (January 4, 1991) by the Chairman of the Milton Keynes Health Authority when he wrote:

That we are becoming a healthier society, bearing less physical pain than hitherto, is a matter for rejoicing. But as Blake said: 'Joy and woe are woven fine.' The woe is evidenced by the ever-growing legions of barely sentient geriatrics existing in institutions throughout the land. In 1952, the Queen sent 200 telegrams to centenarians. In 1989 she sent 1750, and the spiral is in bleak ascent in the decade ahead.

When the cost implications of all this are understood I forecast that, as we now have abortion, virtually on demand, calls for euthanasia to be legalised will become hard to resist.

When a predecessor version of the present chapter was read to the European Association Conference in October 1990, a young lecturer in

Geriatric Medicine from one of the London Teaching Hospitals remarked that he believed the paper identified the major moral issue – the pressure for non-voluntary euthanasia – which he thought his generation of geriatricians would have to cope with.

2 The special and inherent value that human lives possess may be reasonably affirmed in virtue of the radical developmental capacity inherent in the nature of every human being. It is this capacity which makes possible the varied achievements of human beings, and in particular the distinctive achievements of adult humans. But if we value these then we should value all the more the nature which is at the root of them.

That nature is in many cases prevented from achieving a satisfactory development of its characteristic potential, and in many cases an achieved development is overtaken by severe decline. But in neither kind of case is it reasonable to cease to respect the nature which continues to characterise the life of defective human beings.

References

Bliss, M. R. (1990). Resources, the family and voluntary euthanasia. *The British Journal of General Practice*, **40**, 117–122.
Williams, B. (1985). Which slopes are slippery? In *Moral Dilemmas in Modern Medicine*, ed. M. Lockwood, 126–37. Oxford: Oxford University Press.

14

Economics, justice and the value of life: concluding remarks

JOHN FINNIS

I

Among the most serious efforts to settle ethical questions by economic reasoning is the Economic Analysis of Law. Richard Posner, a cultured and sophisticated professor of law at Chicago, led a movement which has undertaken a wide-ranging description and evaluation of legal arrangements in terms of their economic efficiency (maximisation of social wealth, particularly by minimisation of wasted 'transaction costs'). At the movement's zenith, Posner himself proposed that the ethics of wealth maximisation is superior to other aggregative theories of morality, notably utilitarianism, and provides 'a comprehensive and unitary criterion of rights and duties' (Posner 1979, 140). Some of its results – such as that 'people who are very poor . . . count only if they are part of the utility function of someone who has wealth' – do (he conceded) 'grate on modern sensibilities'; but none of its positions or implications, he urged, are 'violently inconsistent with our common moral intuitions' (*ibid.*, 128, 131). Ten years later, and now a high-ranking federal judge, Posner withdrew his claim that Economic Analysis of Law affords an appropriate 'comprehensive criterion' of moral judgment, and conceded that it is open to criticisms which cannot be answered. One may doubt the philosophical depth of his formulation of the deepest criticism: that wealth maximisation's potential for approving slavery is 'contrary to the unshakable moral intuitions of Americans' (Posner 1990, 377). But the reluctant admissions of these ambitious and perceptive theorists are relevant to a reflection on the issues discussed in this book.

Disciplined economic thought is helpful. It brings to light the complexity of the impact which one's choices have, beyond their purpose or intention. It constantly reminds us that to spend on one thing is to use up what might have been spent (time and labour, money, other resources) on other purposes. But it cannot capture the idea of justice or the sense of our purpose to be just and to do justice. For economic thought, as such, cannot comprehend and explain either of the two basic forms of justice's requirements: that one abstain from those types of choice and action which are incompatible with decent, proper, acceptable treatment of another human being; and that one abstain from causing and accepting (let alone intending) unfair consequences, even 'mere' side-effects of one's chosen action and of its intended effects.

The problem with any and every kind of economic reasoning taken as a comprehensive criterion of rational choice is that it seeks the maximisation of value, measuring better and worse, greater good and lesser evil by aggregating units of a single measure of value – what people are willing and able to pay in dollars or dollar equivalents (see Posner 1979, 119–20). But if reason could accomplish such an aggregation – i.e. if the action involving overall aggregate net greatest good were identifiable – *choice*, morally significant and rationally guided election between open alternatives, would be neither necessary nor, strictly speaking, possible. For the alternative courses of action, involving aggregate lesser good, would have *no* rational attraction. In reality, of course, morally significant choices are everywhere open and pressing, precisely because the goods involved, especially the goods fundamental to human persons, cannot be weighed and measured in the way that economics, like every aggregative method proposed for directing choice (e.g. utilitarianism), requires. Such choices involve incommensurables. (Finnis, Boyle & Grisez, 1987, 243–72; Boyle, Grisez & Finnis, 1990.)

By no means all measurements and comparisons relevant to human action are impossible or outside the range of reason. For example, the precise goal of some particular procedure or intervention or administration of drugs provides a rational measure of efficacy and, in that sense, of benefit; some at least of the costs involved in seeking that goal can similarly be rationally assessed by reference to specific measures such as money, or pain imposed compared with pain relieved.

But any full assessment of options in the treatment of elderly long-term-care patients will escape the bounds of measurability. For the irreversible debility and dependence of the patient raises a question, not so much about the physiological benefit or futility of specific treatments, but rather about whether the specific benefit obtainable from any treatment, even the most ordinary and inexpensive, is a benefit which, *all things considered*, is worth seeking and having. Perhaps this patient's continued existence, even with the comfort and sustenance afforded by a meal or a drink, is of no benefit to anyone? What we should think in response to that question is the theme of the next section. My present point concerns the practical context in which the question is a live issue, the context of choice between alternative options.

For: many people have come to think that one should guide one's moral judgment by first identifying one option as promising greater overall net good or less overall net bad than alternative options. But such a calculus of greater pre-moral good and lesser pre-moral bad is impossible (not merely impracticable: impossible) wherever there is a morally significant choice. And the present context well illustrates one of the main sources of this pre-moral incommensurability of options. A first option is to continue to give or accept sustenance. A second option is to withhold or withdraw it, in the belief that the patient's continuing life in itself involves and imposes costs outweighing any benefits obtainable from it and its sustenance; the proposal is to terminate life in order to cut these costs by discontinuing sustenance – in other words, to kill the patient by deliberate omission, omission chosen as a means to an end. A third option is to withhold or withdraw sustenance, on the subtly different ground that giving sustenance is wasteful because the patient's continuing life yields no net benefit; one's purpose again is to minimise costs, and one's proposal is not precisely to kill (as a means of reducing overall costs) but to *abandon* the patient to death (judging that the means of sustaining the patient would better be kept for or devoted to some other purpose). My point, then, is this: the benefits and costs involved in alternative options such as these are real and striking but elude an economic calculus or any other process of aggregating pre-moral goods. Each is an option with enormous implications and ramifications for everyone's life and existence. Whichever proposal is adopted or recommended, the choice (or recommendation) is one which will impact on the character of the chooser (or recommender) and of every potential chooser, on the character of health-care professionals, on the relationship of trust between health-care professionals and their clients, on the attitude of everyone to his or her own body and bodily life, on the whole substance of solidarity between the strong and the weak at all stages of life ... And all these effects quite elude measurement, yet are very real and are really involved, as benefits and harms, in the only relevant object of weighing and comparing: the alternative *options* (of treating/sustaining, of killing, and of abandoning the patient) to be considered in deliberation and accepted or rejected in free choice.

II

To have a just understanding of, and disposition towards, the value of a human being's bodily life, it is not enough to be aware of the fallacies of every economism which would apply a technique (legitimate in resolving technical problems) to non-technical decisions. One of the sternest and most effective critics of Economic Analysis of Law has been Ronald Dworkin, longtime Professor of Jurisprudence at Oxford and now also at New York University. And Dworkin, whose interpretation of liberalism expresses attitudes and policies widely accepted and often applied, has recently taken to affirming what he calls 'the intrinsic value of human life'.

But by this phrase, Dworkin means no more than: 'once a human life has begun it is terribly important that it goes well' (Dworkin 1991, 17). The implication is that there are human lives which are not going, or are likely not to go, 'well enough' to be worth living. Thus the phrase hitherto taken as foundational for the 'pro-life' case against abortion is purloined to convey a meaning from which 'it sometimes follows that abortion is morally recommended or required'. (*ibid.*).

Correspondingly, Dworkin vehemently rejects the view that the life of the comatose has any value: the life of the permanently vegetative is 'not valuable to anyone' (*ibid.*, 15). It is not in their interests to live on, indeed it is plausible or right to think that continuing to live on is, for them, a net disadvantage, and that they are better off dead (*ibid.*, 16). Polishing the similar rhetoric of Justice Stevens of the US Supreme Court, more cautiously shared by the other three dissenting Justices in *Cruzan* v. *Director Missouri Department of Health* 110 Supreme Court Reports 2841 (1990), Dworkin holds: 'There is no way in which continued life can be good for such people'. Indeed, 'it is at least a reasonable view that a permanently comatose person is, for all that matters, dead already'; the 'bodies they used to inhabit' are only 'technically alive'. And: to care for them is to show 'pointless and degrading solicitude' (*ibid.*).

This is not the place to attempt any full unravelling of the ways one's intrinsic dignity is related to and yet not determined by indignities which one may undergo or the undignified aspects of one's dependence in illness, disintegration, dying ... Certainly, a comatose person can be subjected to indignities, e.g. by being treated as a sex object, or by being dumped into the garbage, or by being systematically called a vegetable. But the rhetoric which Dworkin takes over from (dissenting) judgments of Supreme Court Justices is sinister in its systematic confusion of the emotionally repugnant aspects of long-term coma (the mess of excrement and so forth) with lack of human dignity. These distinguished lawyers, offering to speak for the interests of the comatose, shroud these people with epithets calculated to de-humanise them (preparatory, it is to be feared, to justifying the deliberate termination of their lives). So it is said that for such people 'the burden of maintaining the corporeal existence degrades the very human-ity it was meant to serve'; their life is one of degradation; someone on life support has a 'degraded existence' (Brennan J. in *Cruzan*). In short, all such remarks confuse the emotional sense of 'dignity', 'dignified/ undignified', and 'indignity' with the rational and essential sense of 'human dignity'. For in the latter sense it is indeed true to say that one who helps the comatose, or other severely mentally disabled people, is affirming and serving their dignity and expressing solidarity with them as, while gravely disabled, still human persons.

But is such care pointless? Does it at best affirm a value which is absent, and at worst impose on the object of care still further disvalue? Do the unconscious (or other severely mentally disabled persons) who can no longer do good things or have good experiences benefit at all from their continued existence? Does caring for them benefit either them or others? Does it maintain human solidarity with them, or is it just sentimental folly?

If, as Dworkin and Stevens explicitly and Brennan and others implicitly contend, one's life without cognitive-affective function, one's mere physical existence, is of no value, constitutes no benefit, then that bodily life must be merely an instrumental good, something which persons have and use for their specifically human or personal purposes but which remains really distinct from what human persons *are*. One who has only this has ceased to be *as* a person, has *no personal interests* at stake, 'is for all that matters dead already'.

But this is an issue to be decided by reason, not feeling and rhetorically stirred imagination. When one considers living in a coma, one is over-whelmed by the distance between this condition and the integral good of a flourishing human person. Nobody wants to be in that condition; no decent person wants anyone to be in it. The good of human life is *very inadequately* instantiated in such a life, so deprived and so unhealthy. But this does not show that human life considered in abstraction from all other human goods such as play, friendship, awareness of truth and beauty, is of no intrinsic goodness. *No* human good, considered *apart from* all the others, in a mode of existence (if it were possible) deprived of all the others, is appealing. But this does not show that basic human goods, such as those I have just mentioned, are instrumental, or other than intrinsically good. No more does the unappealing nature of comatose life show it to be valueless. For it is the very actuality of one's living body, and one's living body is one's person.

To deny that one's living body is one's person is to accept some sort of dualistic theory of human persons, according to which human beings are inherently disembodied realities who only *have* their bodies, only inhabit them and use them. (This is clearly the basis on which Stevens J. proceeds in *Cruzan's* case: unconscious, therefore not a person, *therefore* not really living.)

No form of dualism is rationally defensible. For every dualism sets out to be a theory of one's personal identity as a unitary and subsisting self – a self always organically living but only discontinuously conscious, and now and then inquiring and judging, deliberating and choosing, and employing techniques and instruments to achieve purposes. But every form of dualism renders inexplicable the unity in complexity which one experiences in every act one consciously does. We experience this (complex) unity more intimately and thoroughly than any other unity in the world; indeed, it is for us the very paradigm of substantial unity and identity. As I write this, I am the unitary subject of my fingers hitting the keys, the sensations I feel in them, the thinking I am articulating, my commitment to write this paper, my use of the computer to express myself. So the one reality that I am involves at once consciousness and bodily behaviour; and dualism sets out to explain *me*. 'But every dualism ends by denying that there is any *one* something of which to be the theory. It does not explain *me*; it tells me about two things, one a nonbodily person and the other a nonpersonal body, neither of which I can recognise as myself.' (Grisez 1990, 37; see also Finnis *et al.*, 1987, 304–9; Finnis 1989, 267–8.)

So, one's living body is intrinsic to one's personal reality. One does not merely possess, inhabit or use one's body, as one possesses and uses an instrument or inhabits a dwelling. Thus, human life, which is nothing other than the very actuality of one's body, is a good intrinsic to one. It is not merely an instrumental good of the person, or extrinsic to the person. Intrinsic to the original unity of the person, it shares in the dignity of the person.

Like other basic, intrinsic human goods, human bodily life can be instantiated more or less perfectly. When instantiated most perfectly, it includes vital functions such as speech, deliberation and free choice; then it is most obviously proper to the person. But even an impoverished instantiation of the good of life remains specifically human and proper to the person whose life it is. Human life is inherently good, and does not cease to be good when one can no longer enjoy a degree of cognitive-affective function or attain other values. Human bodily life, even the life of one in a coma, has value. To choose to kill even such a person is to choose to harm that person. It is therefore inconsistent with a rational love of that person, and (however much motivated by feelings of affection and compassed about with thoughts and words of respect) is inconsistent with respect for and justice to the person. Whatever the feelings of solidarity which may accompany and suggest such a choice, it is a choice incompatible with a reasonable solidarity with the person so killed.

Such a choice differs radically from two other sorts of choice or attitude with which euthanasiasts usually confuse it. (i) Whereas the choice to confer relief from suffering or embarrassment ('indignity') or expense *by* killing (by action or omission) is a choice to impose harm *to the whole* person *as a means* (of benefiting the person), the choice to remove a diseased organ or limb in order to save the patient is not a choice of *harm to the person* at all. (*Contra* McCormick 1981, 647; on McCormick's analysis of amputation Daniel Maguire builds the ethical theory of 'proportionate reason' which he employs to defend and advocate euthanasia: Maguire (1975), 71, 126.) What is and is not harming is to be judged by reference to the whole person whose organically integral bodily well-being is the reason for choosing to remove the diseased part, not by reference to the part whose disease threatens that organic integration nor by reference to any part which is damaged as an unavoidable side-effect of the treatment. Therapeutic surgery is not a case of choosing to do harm (or any other sort of evil) for the sake of good. (ii) The choice not to undergo further medical treatment, because of its expense, riskiness, painfulness or other burdens, can be a reasonable choice even in cases where it is known that the consequence of the choice will be an early death. Here death is not sought as a means (still less as an end), but is simply accepted as a side-effect.

Such an acceptance need not be based on any attempt (which would be doomed to failure) to evaluate continued life as valueless, or as objectively less valuable than relief from expense, risk, pain or other burdens. It may be based simply on aversion to the burdens or costs of the treatment. These are burdens or costs which rational deliberation can take into account; they provide reasons for forgoing the treatment. But in situations of morally significant choice, as I have already stressed, reasons constituted by costs and burdens cannot be measured by aggregating them for comparison with ('weighing' against) net benefits. Deliberating will come down, instead, to a matter of one's personal response to the competing reasons. One's deliberation should set aside *merely* emotional motivations such as feelings of anxiety. But it will not exclude one's affective response to the relevant reasons.

The feelings involved in such an affective response are not themselves required or shaped by reason. Nor, in someone of upright character, will they be contrary to reason. But every choice of (intention to do) harm to the person will be contrary to reason because contrary to a reason (e.g. 'the basic human good of life and health is to be pursued and respected') which cannot be rationally outweighed. So, whatever one's feelings, it cannot be right to intend death or any other harm to oneself or another. It can be reasonable to act on one's aversion to the costs and benefits, provided one is not making a choice contrary to any of the rational requirements which we call moral standards. These standards include not only the norm excluding intent to kill or harm, and the norm requiring fairness to others (e.g. one's children or others dependent upon one's continued life and activity), but also highly specific standards which one has made relevant to oneself by one's commitments, vocation and particular undertakings. (This paragraph does no more than sketch some essentials; for a much fuller and more nuanced discussion, involving similar principles and judgments, see Grisez 1990.)

III

Talk of maintaining solidarity with and fidelity to the very dependent can sound vague and high falutin', not to say abstract and fishy. But the papers of the health-care professionals in this collection – particularly those of Graham Mulley, Marion Hildick-Smith and Robert Stout – convey something of solidarity's practical substance and realism. The considerations and measures they advance are relatively simple and straightforward (though they certainly call for imagination and sympathy). But these considerations and measures are the working out of an attitude which classical philosophy and theology called *general justice*: an all-round decency of individuals both in their individual capacities and as making decisions on behalf of a community (whether at the level of hospital, local authority, or central government).

As for fairness – that rational standard whose particular content is, however, dependent upon feelings and other contingencies – its requirements cut both ways. Politically demanding and effective groups of the elderly can propose and secure the placing of unjustifiable burdens on younger persons with immediate responsibility for children; levels of pensions, and arrangements about house ownership, for example, can in some modern Western democracies impose unfair burdens in the interests of the elderly. But that should not distract us from the very real concerns ventilated in the papers of Michael Banner, Joseph Boyle and Luke Gormally. And John Keown's survey of the emergence and wildfire spread of euthanasia in the Netherlands provides us with a striking example of the downward spiral in which an irrational attitude to human bodily life (treating an intrinsic and basic good as if it were extrinsic and instrumental) reinforces and is reinforced by an irrational belief in the possibility of rationally aggregating the costs and benefits involved in the alternative options: (a) killing out of compassion, and (b) care which excludes both the choice to kill (by act or omission) and the choice to continue treatment which is futile or imposes burdens one has no responsibility in fairness or fortitude to bear.

Some questions of allocation or rationing of resources are easy to make, as Robert Stout suggests. Others will always remain difficult questions, about which reasonable people will reasonably disagree with each other, making different and incompatible choices within the range of not unreasonable options. But some problems of allocation or rationing will remain questions which we can and should answer prior to all reasonably disputable issues of allocation, and which we can and should answer in a definite direction, thereby establishing boundaries for all subsequent allocative choices. Luke Gormally indicates one of these boundaries:

> ... what is *minimally required* in the provision of health care for the debilitated elderly is a quality of care which so far as possible reduces the temptation to doctors, nurses and others to think that they would do better to kill some of their patients rather than provide them with manifestly inadequate care, i.e. care of a kind which leads to rapid deterioration or which fails to palliate. The inadequate care of patients creates the temptation to dispose of patients who are obviously held in low esteem. By contrast, adequate care signifies that the patients are valued.

This, of course, identifies what is 'minimally required' in a well-resourced society; there can be social conditions where no treatment actually available prevents rapid deterioration or succeeds in palliating distress, and where what care and sustenance is available is fairly reserved for the young. But even in such conditions, which are far from the conditions of our society, justice excludes all choices to kill, and reason undercuts every claim that the life of the dependent elderly is a null or negative value which one may reasonably choose to terminate.

References

Boyle, J. M., Grisez, G. G. & Finnis, J. M. (1990). Incoherence and consequentialism (or proportionalism) – a rejoinder. *American Catholic Philosophical Quarterly* **64** (1990) 271–7.

Dworkin, R. M. (1991). The right to death. *New York Review of Books*, January 31, 1991, 14–17.

Finnis, J. M. (1989). Persons and their associations. *Proceedings of the Aristotelian Society, Supplementary Volume* **63** (1989) 267–74.

Finnis, J. M., Boyle, J. M. & Grisez, G. G. (1987). *Nuclear Deterrence, Morality and Realism*. Oxford and New York: Clarendon Press.

Grisez, G. G. (1990). Should nutrition and hydration be provided to permanently comatose, and other mentally disabled persons? *Linacre Quarterly*, May 1990, 30–43.

McCormick, Richard A., SJ (1981). *Notes on Moral Theology 1965 through 1980*. Lanham, Maryland: University Press of America.

Maguire, Daniel C. (1975). *Death by Choice*. New York: Schocken Books.

Posner, R. A. (1979). Utilitarianism, economics, and legal theory. *Journal of Legal Studies*, **8**, 103–40.

Posner, R. A. (1990). *The Problems of Jurisprudence*. Cambridge, Massachusetts, and London: Harvard University Press.

Index